Glia Cells and Their Role in Maintenance, Protection, and Development of the Central Nervous System

Edited by
María Elena Hernández Aguilar,
Jorge Manzo and Hugo Manuel Libreros Jiménez

Published in London, United Kingdom

Glia Cells and Their Role in Maintenance, Protection, and Development of the Central Nervous System
http://dx.doi.org/10.5772/intechopen.1009052
Edited by María Elena Hernández Aguilar, Jorge Manzo and Hugo Manuel Libreros Jiménez

Contributors
Elena Puerta, Hugo Manuel Libreros-Jimenez, Inga Zerr, Jorge Manzo-Denes, Julie Pilon, Lamia Bouslama-Oueghlani, Lilesh Kumar Pradhan, Maider Garmendia-Berges, María Elena Hernández-Aguilar, Saima Zafar, Urwah Rasheed, Xiang Gao

First published in London, United Kingdom, 2026 by IntechOpen
IntechOpen is the global imprint of INTECHOPEN LIMITED, registered in England and Wales, registration number: 11086078, 167-169 Great Portland Street, London, W1W 5PF, United Kingdom

For EU product safety concerns: IN TECH d.o.o., Prolaz Marije Krucifikse Kozulić 3, 51000 Rijeka, Croatia, info@intechopen.com or visit our website at intechopen.com.

British Library Cataloguing-in-Publication Data
A catalogue record for this book is available from the British Library

Glia Cells and Their Role in Maintenance, Protection, and Development of the Central Nervous System
Edited by María Elena Hernández Aguilar, Jorge Manzo and Hugo Manuel Libreros Jiménez
p. cm.
Print ISBN 978-1-83769-419-8
Online ISBN 978-1-83769-418-1
eBook (PDF) ISBN 978-1-83769-420-4

If disposing of this product, please recycle the paper responsibly.

Meet the editors

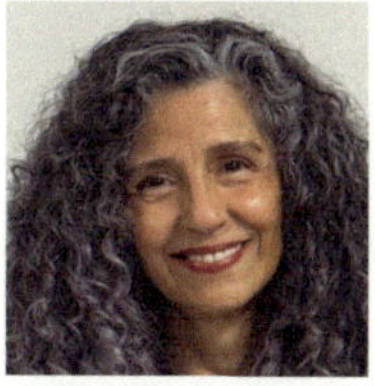

Professor Dr. María Elena Hernández Aguilar works at the Brain Research Institute, Universidad Veracruzana, Xalapa, Veracruz, México. She received her BSc in Biology from Universidad Veracruzana, México, and her MSc and Ph.D. from the Universidad Nacional Autónoma de México in 1993 and 1997, respectively. Her research concentrates on molecular mechanisms involved in prostate cancer. She also investigates how the major pelvic ganglia may be involved in the generation of prostate cancer when neurons have degenerated. She coordinates Ph.D. theses in brain research studies and teaches neuroinmmmunoendocrinology to Ph.D. students. She is a member of the Southeastern Mexican chapter of the Society for Neuroscience and the Mexican Society of Urogenital Sciences. Dr. Aguilar is the recipient of the 2021 State Science and Technology Award.

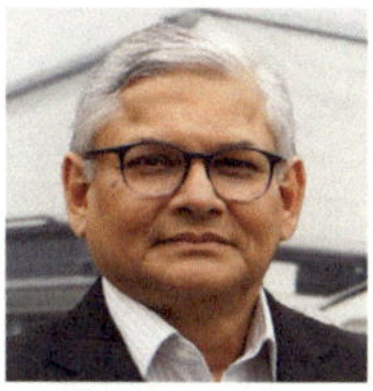

Dr. Jorge Manzo is a neuroscientist at the Brain Research Institute of Universidad Veracruzana (UV), Mexico. He earned his undergraduate degree in Biology from UV, a Master's degree in Reproductive Biology from the Universidad Autónoma de Tlaxcala, and a Ph.D. in Physiological Sciences from the Universidad Nacional Autónoma de México (UNAM). His primary research focus is on the neurobiology of autism spectrum disorder (ASD). By integrating animal models and clinical studies in children, he investigates the neural mechanisms that underlie atypical sensory processing, altered social behavior, and neurodevelopmental disruptions associated with ASD. His earlier work in reproductive neuroendocrinology has contributed to understanding the hormonal regulation of brain and behavior. Dr. Manzo has directed numerous undergraduate, master's, and doctoral theses, and is a recipient of the Veracruz State Prize in Science and Technology. In 2024, he was named Decano by Universidad Veracruzana.

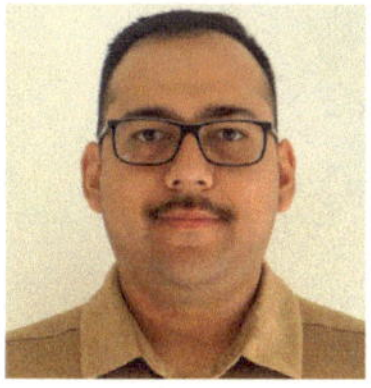

Hugo M. Libreros Jiménez holds a degree in Mechatronics Engineering from the Instituto Tecnológico Superior de Xalapa and a Ph.D. in Brain Research from the Universidad Veracruzana. His career combines industrial experience in telecommunications and neuroscience research, particularly in Autism Spectrum Disorder, brain-machine interfaces, and neurotechnology. He has actively participated in scientific outreach and presented his work at national and International conferences. He is currently a Postdoctoral Research Associate in the Regenerative Neurobiology and Neuroelectronics Laboratory at the University of Arizona (2026), focusing on microelectrode technologies for recording brain and peripheral activity in amputation and hypertension models. His current project explores neurointerfaces for motor control and sensory feedback in bionic limbs. He is the author of the article "On the Cranial Nerves" (NeuroSci, 2024) and was recently elected as an associate member for 2025 by Sigma Xi, "The Scientific Research Honor Society".

Contents

Preface

Glia Cells and Their Role in Maintenance, Protection, and Development of the Central Nervous System is a specialized work that invites the readers to reexamine the role of glial cells through a contemporary lens. For decades, neuroscience focused predominantly on neurons and neural stem cells as the primary drivers of neurogenesis. However, growing evidence indicates that glial cells not only accompany these processes but also actively shape the generation, maturation, and functionality of new neurons in both the developing and the adult brain.

This book arises from the need to integrate the dispersed, often underestimated knowledge of the dynamic interplay between glial cells and neurogenic processes. Throughout its chapters, the reader will find an updated and comprehensive view of how astrocytes, microglia, radial glia, and oligodendrocytes contribute to neuronal proliferation, differentiation, and integration. The volume also explores the mechanisms by which glial cells influence brain plasticity, tissue repair, and the progression of neurological diseases.

Its structure combines insights from molecular biology, physiology, developmental neurobiology, and clinical neuroscience, offering a multidisciplinary and accessible panorama for both specialists and advanced students. Each chapter provides conceptual and experimental elements that help elucidate how glia create, modulate, and safeguard the neural environment, and why their study is essential for the design of regenerative therapies and clinical interventions.

We hope this book will serve as a valuable reference for the biomedical community interested in the cellular foundations of neurogenesis and its implications for brain health. We trust that readers will find here a solid starting point for delving deeper into a rapidly evolving field, where glial cells—at last—take their rightful place at the center of nervous system biology.

Finally, we extend our sincere appreciation to all the contributors whose work made this volume possible, and to the IntechOpen team for their kind invitation and support throughout the development of this project.

María Elena Hernández-Aguilar,
Jorge Manzo-Denes and Hugo Manuel Libreros-Jimenez
Brain Research Institute,
Universidad Veracruzana,
Xalapa, Veracruz, México

Section 1

Introduction

Chapter 1

Introductory Chapter: Glial Cells and Their Role in the Maintenance, Protection, and Development of the Central Nervous System

María Elena Hernández-Aguilar, Jorge Manzo-Denes and Hugo Manuel Libreros-Jimenez

1. Overview of glial cells

The term glia derives from the Greek γλία, meaning glue, bond, or adhesive, and refers to a heterogeneous group of cells with specialized functions. Glial cells are a fundamental component of the central nervous system (CNS) and exist in proportions comparable to neurons. Although it was long believed that glia outnumber neurons by a ratio of 10 to 1, current evidence indicates that both populations are present in approximately equal numbers [1].

For decades, glial cells were viewed primarily as structural and metabolic support for neurons. However, advances in microscopy, molecular biology, and transcriptomics have revealed that glia actively contribute to homeostasis, neural plasticity, and the defense of nervous tissue.

Glia include astrocytes, oligodendrocytes, microglia, and ependymal cells. Each population possesses distinct morphological and functional characteristics that collectively sustain the physiological integrity of the neural microenvironment. Understanding their structure and function in physiological contexts is essential for elucidating mechanisms underlying neurodegenerative diseases [1].

2. Maintenance of neural homeostasis

2.1 Astrocytes

Astrocytes are characterized by their numerous processes, which give them a star-like appearance and inspire their name. They are the most abundant and versatile glial cell type in the CNS. Astrocytes regulate cerebral blood flow, recycle neurotransmitters, supply glucose to neurons, and support synaptic plasticity.

They also maintain extracellular ion and neurotransmitter balance, preventing excitotoxicity, and modulate synaptic communication. Additionally, they are integral components of the blood–brain barrier. Through extensive processes, astrocytes form close contacts with blood vessels and can increase blood flow to

IntechOpen

regions of elevated neuronal activity. Their simultaneous interactions with neurons enable the integration of metabolic and electrical signals. Consequently, astrocytes influence not only synaptic plasticity but also learning and memory processes [1].

2.2 Oligodendrocytes

The term oligodendrocyte derives from the Greek words oligo (small), dendro (tree), and cyto (cell), collectively meaning "small tree-like cell." These cells produce the myelin sheath that insulates axons and are essential for maintaining CNS homeostasis. This multilaminar sheath permits the electrical isolation of axons and supports saltatory conduction, increasing conduction velocity and energy efficiency.

Oligodendrocytes are distributed throughout the CNS, with a higher density in white matter. Although their principal role is myelination, they also contribute to microenvironmental stability and tissue repair. Recent studies reveal that oligodendrocytes maintain dynamic interactions with the axons they ensheath, respond to changes in neuronal activity, and possess limited regenerative capacity. Consequently, myelin deterioration or oligodendrocyte loss is associated with disorders such as multiple sclerosis, metabolic diseases, and genetically mediated demyelinating conditions [2–4].

3. Protection and immune response in the CNS

3.1 Microglia

Microglia are the resident immune cells of the CNS and share structural and functional similarities with tissue macrophages. They are the least abundant CNS cell population. Derived from the myeloid lineage during embryonic development, microglia continually survey neural tissue for signs of damage, pathogens, or disruptions in homeostasis. When exposed to harmful stimuli, they adopt a reactive phenotype, altering their morphology and releasing pro- and anti-inflammatory interleukins.

Beyond their defensive functions, microglia participate in synaptic pruning, a critical process for establishing functional neuronal circuits. They also phagocytose apoptotic cells, cellular debris, and aberrant proteins. These activities persist throughout life, facilitating the refinement of synaptic networks and the maintenance of normal CNS function. Furthermore, microglia contribute to angiogenesis and express both the common leukocyte antigen and class II major histocompatibility complex molecules, which are typical of antigen-presenting cells. They also possess receptors for glutamate and GABA [5–7].

3.2 Ependymal cells

Ependymal cells line the brain ventricles and the ependymal canal and include several morphologically distinct subtypes. Ciliated ependymal cells are typically cuboidal, whereas tanycytes exhibit elongated cell bodies and specialized contact with neural tissue. A third, less abundant subtype – radial ependymal cells – shares morphological traits with other ependymal cells but possesses a long basal process. These radial cells are found at the dorsal or ventral poles of the ependymal layer, with basal processes oriented along the dorsoventral axis.

Their functions include regulating cerebrospinal fluid (CSF) flow, transporting molecules, and contributing to neurogenic niches. Their strategic anatomical position facilitates communication between the CSF and brain parenchyma, influencing waste clearance, inflammatory responses, and homeostasis of the internal environment [8–10].

4. The silent revolution of glial cells

Over the past decade, the study of glia has transformed from a peripheral area of interest into a central pillar of contemporary neuroscience. This volume invites readers to reconsider long-standing assumptions about the brain. Rather than being a simple collection of chapters, it offers an entry point into the intersection of neuroscience, immunology, developmental biology, molecular biology, physiology, and medicine.

It is designed for students, academics, clinicians, and researchers seeking to understand not only what glial cells are, but what they do – and why their study is essential for understanding the principles underlying neuroglia and anticipating the advances that will shape the future of the field.

A comprehensive understanding of glia–neuron dynamics is fundamental not only for deciphering nervous system physiology but also for developing novel therapeutic strategies for disorders such as Alzheimer's disease, amyotrophic lateral sclerosis, epilepsy, autism, and others.

Author details

María Elena Hernández-Aguilar[1*], Jorge Manzo-Denes[1] and Hugo Manuel Libreros-Jimenez[2]

1 Institute of Brain Research, Veracruzana University, Xalapa, Mexico

2 PhD in Brain Research, Veracruzana University, Xalapa, Mexico

*Address all correspondence to: elenahernandez@uv.mx

References

[1] Allen NJ, Lyons DA. Glia as architects of central nervous system formation and function. Science. 2018;**362**(6411):181–185. DOI: 10.1126/science.aat0473

[2] Barres BA. The mystery and magic of glia: A perspective on their roles in health and disease. Neuron. 2008;**60**(3):430–440. DOI: 10.1016/j.neuron.2008.10.013

[3] Fields RD. A new mechanism of nervous system plasticity: Activity-dependent myelination. Nature Reviews Neuroscience. 2015;**16**(12):756–767. DOI: 10.1038/nrn4023

[4] Noori R, Park D, Griffiths JD, Bells S, Frankland PW, Mabbott D, Lefebvre JS. Activity-dependent myelination: A glial mechanism of oscillatory self-organization in large-scale brain networks. Proceedings of the National Academy of Sciences USA. 2020;**117**(24):13227–13237. DOI: 10.1073/pnas.1916646117

[5] Kettenmann H, Hanisch U-K, Noda M, Verkhratsky A. Physiology of microglia. Physiological Reviews. 2021;**101**(2):1347–1421. DOI: 10.1152/physrev.00011.2020

[6] Gao C, Jiang J, Tan Y, Chen S. Microglia in neurodegenerative diseases: mechanism and potential therapeutic targets. Signal Transduction and Targeted Therapy. 2023;**8**(1):359. DOI: 10.1038/s41392-023-01588-0

[7] Prinz M, Jung S, Priller J. Microglia Biology: One Century of Evolving Concepts. Cell. 2019;**179**(2, 3):292–311. DOI: 10.1016/j.cell.2019.08.053

[8] Deng S, Gan L, Xu T, Zhou S, Zhang Z, Yang GY, Tian H, Tang Y. Roles of Ependymal Cells in the Physiology and Pathology of the Central Nervous System. Aging and Disease. 2023;**14**(2):468–483. DOI: 10.14336/AD.2022.0826-1

[9] Lacroix S, Hamilton LK, Vaugeois A, Beaudoin S, Breault-Dugas C, Pineau I, Lévesque SA, Grégoire CA, Fernandes KJL. Central canal ependymal cells proliferate extensively in response to traumatic spinal cord injury but not demyelinating lesions. PLoS ONE. 2014;**9**(1):e85916. DOI: 10.1371/journal.pone.0085916

[10] Meletis K, Barnabé-Heider F, Carlén M, Evergren E, Tomilin N, Shupliakov O, Frisén J. Spinal cord injury reveals multilineage differentiation of ependymal cells. PLoS Biology. 2008;**6**(7):e182. DOI: 10.1371/journal.pbio.0060182

Section 2

Microglia as Regulators of Neuronal Microenvironment

Chapter 2

Microglia: Key Players in Perineuronal Net Dynamics

Maider Garmendia-Berges and Elena Puerta

Abstract

Perineuronal nets (PNNs) are specialized extracellular matrix structures in the central nervous system that selectively enwrap certain neuronal populations. They have a highly organized structure that progressively forms during neurodevelopment, coinciding in time with the closure of critical periods of heightened plasticity. In fact, PNNs are involved in the regulation of neuronal plasticity and, therefore, regulate higher processes such as memory. They also have a protective role on the neurons they surround, further underscoring their importance. Notably, PNN disruptions have been observed in several pathological conditions, rendering their regulation potentially valuable. Among the factors that modulate PNNs, microglia stand out for their relevance. These cells alter PNNs through phagocytosis of their components and the release of proteolytic enzymes, which seems to gain significance during neurodevelopment and pathological conditions. This chapter focuses on PNNs, their structure, function, and role under physiological and pathological conditions, emphasizing the relevance of microglia in regulating their dynamics.

Keywords: extracellular matrix, microglia, neurological disorders, neurodevelopment, neuronal activity, perineuronal nets

1. Introduction

All structures in the Central Nervous System (CNS) are embedded in the extracellular matrix (ECM), which constitutes approximately 20% of the brain volume [1]. Besides providing structural support, the ECM is essential for maintaining brain homeostasis, as it interacts directly or through ligands to regulate higher functions such as cell proliferation, migration, neuronal activity, and synaptic plasticity. In fact, in the tetrapartite synapse model proposed by Dityatev and Rusakov [2], the ECM represents one of the four elements that interact to enable synaptic plasticity, along with pre- and post-synaptic terminals and glial cells.

Most of the ECM in the brain forms a diffuse and homogeneous network known as the interstitial matrix. However, it also gives rise to structurally and functionally diverse compartments, such as basement membranes, perinodal matrix, and perineuronal nets (PNNs) [3].

PNNs are compact and specialized ECM structures that enwrap certain neuronal subsets, surrounding their soma, axonal initial segment, and proximal dendrites. First described by Camillo Golgi in 1893, PNNs remain a topic of scientific interest, as abnormalities in these structures are closely linked to aging and a range of neurological disorders, including Alzheimer's disease (AD) [4, 5], Parkinson's disease (PD) [6], schizophrenia [7], autism spectrum disorder (ASD) [8, 9] and epilepsy [10]. These pathological alterations include changes in PNN number and density, preferential accumulation around certain populations, and delays in their appearance (for a review, see [11]). Over the last decades, significant progress has been made in characterizing and understanding their structure, functions, and dynamics; however, the key factors regulating their formation and degradation, as well as the different cell types involved in these processes, are still under active investigation. In this regard, the present chapter will particularly compile and analyze the current evidence supporting the role of microglia, the innate immune cells of the CNS, in the regulation of PNNs.

2. Perineuronal nets

2.1. Structure and distribution

PNNs have a highly organized honeycomb-like structure with four primary components: (1) hyaluronan and its synthesizing enzymes, hyaluronan synthases (HAS); (2) members of the Chondroitin Sulfate Proteoglycans (CSPGs) family; (3) hyaluronan- and proteoglycan-binding link proteins, such as Hapln1 and Hapln4; and (4) tenascins (Tn–C and Tn–R). Hyaluronan, the most abundant and essential component of PNNs, is attached to the neuronal surface and forms the backbone of the net, to which CSPGs attach via Hapln1 and Hapln4. Tenascins, in turn, interact with CSPGs and create cross-links, being essential for PNN assembly [12]. Among the main structural features that distinguish PNNs from the diffuse ECM is the greater presence of CSPGs. These proteoglycans vary in their core protein and the amount, length, and type of covalently linked glycosaminoglycan (GAG) side chains, resulting in five CSPG family members: aggrecan, brevican, neurocan, versican, and phosphacan [12] (**Figure 1**).

PNNs undergo continuous turnover and remodeling, a dynamic process tightly regulated by a variety of enzymes released by both neurons and glial cells. Among the molecular regulators of PNN formation, the homeoprotein Otx2 stands out as a transcription factor that promotes PNN accumulation by binding to GAG chains in parvalbumin-expressing GABAergic interneurons (PV neurons) [13]. Other molecules, such as semaphorin 3A and neuronal pentraxin 2, have also been implicated in promoting PNN assembly [14–16]. In contrast, PNN degradation is primarily mediated by extracellular proteases, including MMPs, plasmin, and members of the ADAMTS family (a disintegrin and metalloproteinase with thrombospondin motifs) [12]. The activity of these enzymes is further modulated by regulatory proteins such as TIMPs, tissue-type plasminogen activator (tPA), and plasminogen activator inhibitor [17], ensuring a balanced remodeling of the ECM surrounding neurons.

PNNs present a heterogeneous distribution and abundance throughout the CNS. They mostly enwrap fast-spiking PV neurons [18–20], but not exclusively. PNNs

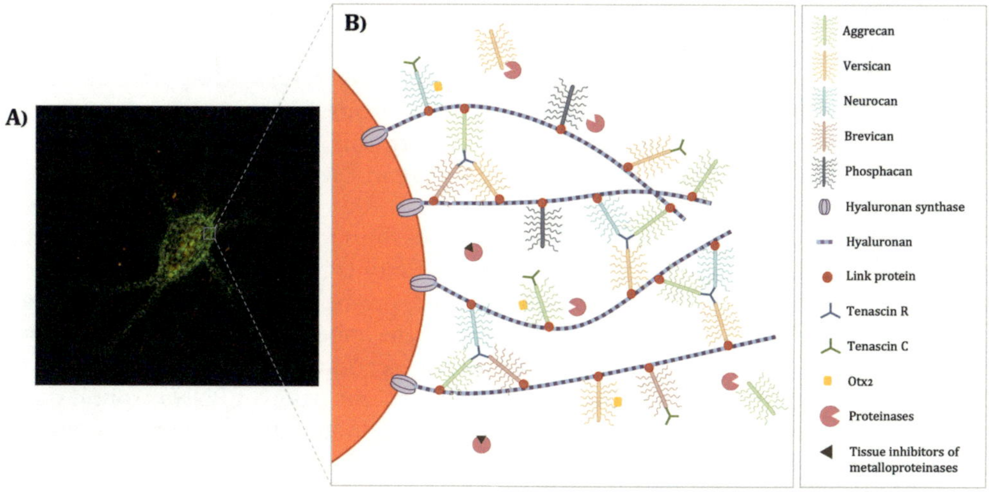

Figure 1.
Structure of a perineuronal net (PNN). (A) Inmunohistochemistry image of a parvalbumin positive interneuron (orange) surrounded by a PNN (green) in mouse cortex. PNN staining was performed using wisteria floribunda agglutinin, which specifically binds to N-acetylgalactosamine residues of chondroitin sulfate proteoglycans (CSPG). (B) PNNs have a hyaluronan backbone that is tied to the neuronal surface through the hyaluronan synthase. Link proteins (Hapln1 and Hapln4) create bonds between hyaluronan and five members of the CSPG family: aggrecan, versican, neurocan, brevican, and phosphacan. The CSPGs form cross-links through tenascins. The degradation of the PNN is mostly carried out by matrix metalloproteinases (MMPs) while tissue inhibitors of metalloproteinases (TIMPs) limit their activity. In turn, Otx2 binds to CSPGs to promote PNN accumulation.

also sparsely form around other inhibitory and excitatory cells in the brain and spinal cord [21–24] and pyramidal CA2 neurons [25]. In the cerebellar cortex, PNNs can be found around Lugaro cells [26] and Golgi GABAergic interneurons [27], and in the deep cerebellar nuclei around excitatory and inhibitory neurons [28].

2.2. Functions

2.2.1. Regulation of neuronal plasticity and memory

PNNs progressively aggregate during postnatal development, and their appearance around some PV neurons aligns in time with the closure of the critical periods (CPs) of heightened plasticity. CPs are windows of maximal cortical plasticity during the early development of the brain that open at different times depending on the region. These windows begin when local inhibitory circuits start to mature, and PV neurons gradually become enwrapped by PNNs. CPs are experience-dependent; sensory inputs are necessary to refine neural circuits in response to environmental stimuli and to promote PNN formation [29–31]. Once PV neurons are fully mature and completely surrounded by PNNs, the CP closes, and plasticity remains thereafter restricted, limiting cognitive flexibility and consolidating the retention of learning experiences and long-term memory [32]. Studies show that juvenile plasticity is recovered in adult rats when PNNs are degraded either by Hapln1 knockout [33] or by treatment with chondroitinase ABC (ch-ABC), which degrades PNNs by cleaving GAG side chains of CSPGs

[34–36]. The presence of PNNs in the hippocampal CA2 region further illustrates their role in limiting synaptic plasticity. This area is molecularly distinct from other hippocampal subfields and is characterized by its lack of plasticity. PNNs surrounding CA2 pyramidal neurons and their excitatory synapses restrict their plasticity. Consistent with this, enzymatic disruption of PNNs by ch-ABC enables long-term potentiation in CA2, which is typically absent in this region [25].

One of the most compelling pieces of evidence supporting the key role of PNNs in the opening and closure of CPs of synaptic plasticity is the function of the homeoprotein Otx2, which, as mentioned above, promotes PNN formation around PV interneurons. In fact, the experience-dependent import of Otx2 into PV cells sets the onset of a CP [37, 38]. As Otx2 progressively accumulates in PV neurons, it promotes their maturation and the concomitant accumulation of PNNs around them. A positive feedback loop takes place between PNN condensation and Otx2 retention, such that, once PNNs are completely formed, Otx2 transfer remains constant to maintain the closure of the CP [39]. Remarkably, the loss of Otx2 in adulthood is sufficient to disrupt PNNs and reactivate juvenile-like plasticity [13], further supporting its pivotal role in the regulation of PNNs and cortical plasticity.

Another factor that influences PNN function and its implication on neuronal activity is the sulfation pattern of the CSPGs that compose it, which differs across life stages [32]. They can be sulfated in the 4 (4S) or 6 (6S) carbon position, or disulfated in the 2,6 and 4,6 positions, which define their charge distribution and binding properties. The 4S form is more restrictive to synaptic plasticity, while the 6S form is more permissive. In fact, an increase in the 4S/6S ratio is necessary for Otx2 accumulation during development and leads to the termination of plasticity during development, while 6S makes it persist [40]. In addition, the 6S form is more permissive for axonal regeneration [41], while the 4S restricts axonal guidance and growth [42].

Collectively, these observations support the view that PNNs regulate neural plasticity through several complementary mechanisms that operate both structurally and biochemically. Specifically, it has been hypothesized that PNNs limit plasticity via three main processes [43, 44]: (1) limiting the formation of new neuronal contacts [27, 45, 46], (2) acting as a scaffold where molecules that affect synaptic activity bind [14, 47], and (3) restricting receptor mobility at synapses [48].

Since memory relies on activity-dependent synaptic plasticity, researchers have also investigated whether changes in PNNs can affect the formation and persistence of different types of memory. Indeed, PNNs play an important role in learning and memory processes throughout life, although their effects are highly cell- and region-specific. For example, the formation and storage of fear memories are impaired when PNNs are removed from brain areas such as the hippocampus, medial prefrontal cortex (PFC), or basolateral amygdala [49, 50], as well as in animals lacking aggrecan in PV neurons across the brain [51]. Disruption of PNNs has also been shown to compromise social memory, as evidenced in mice lacking aggrecan selectively in CA2 pyramidal neurons [51] or following ablation of 4S sulfation, deficits that can be reversed when PNNs or 4S sulfation are restored [52].

In contrast, in other contexts, PNN ablation can facilitate memory performance. For instance, the loss of aggrecan restores PV neuron plasticity in the visual cortex and enhances object recognition memory [53]. Similarly, both Hapln1 knockout and ch-ABC treatment improve long-term object recognition memory and facilitate long-term depression in the perirhinal cortex [54]. Notably, the enhancement in memory observed after ch-ABC treatment diminishes over time, suggesting that as PNNs regenerate, they gradually re-establish their control over plasticity levels.

2.2.2. Buffering function and protection against oxidative stress

PNNs have negative charges that form a polyanionic environment around the neurons they enwrap [55]. The anionic charge density reversibly accumulates cationic molecules, which could act as an immobilized ion exchanger, inducing local molecular gradients of cations such as Ca^{2+}, K^{+}, or Na^{+} [56–58]. This buffering property might enhance the excitability and synchrony of fast-spiking neurons [36, 59].

This ion-trapping property might also be responsible for the neuroprotective effect of PNNs against external stressors. Morawski and colleagues [60] proposed that PNNs play a protective role against oxidative stress after observing that neurons surrounded by PNNs in the human cortex exhibited lipofuscin accumulation less frequently compared to those lacking a net. This neuroprotective function was further supported by findings showing that PNN-enwrapped neurons exhibit lower degeneration in response to iron-induced oxidative stress than non-ensheathed neurons [61], meaning that PNNs confer protection against iron-mediated cell death. This protective effect is highly dependent on key structural components of the net, such as aggrecan, link protein, and Tn–R, highlighting the importance of the intact PNN architecture [62]. In addition, a higher density of PNNs around PV neurons correlates with reduced intracellular oxidative stress, as evidenced by lower levels of DNA oxidation products. Conversely, enzymatic degradation of PNNs increases neuronal susceptibility to oxidative damage [63].

3. PNNs in pathological conditions

In recent years, PNN disturbances have been associated with several neurological diseases and may be of physiological relevance to their etiology and symptoms, therefore representing a potential therapeutic target.

Some alterations in PNN number and intensity have been reported in human postmortem brains of schizophrenic patients. Studies have revealed reduced PNN density in the PFC [64], amygdala, and entorhinal cortex [65], and decreased PV and PNN intensity in the dorsolateral PFC, suggesting lower levels of PV protein and PNN components [66]. Studies carried out in a ketamine-induced schizophrenia mouse model and a double-hit mouse model reproduced these findings, revealing a reduction in the number of PNNs and PV neurons surrounded by PNNs in the medial PFC [7, 67]. In a different schizophrenia mouse model that lacks Gclm (a glutamate-cysteine ligase modifier subunit) and therefore has compromised glutathione synthesis and increased susceptibility to oxidative stress, the authors described a decrease in PNN and PV cells across the brain during development [68]. These anomalies could be functionally relevant in the pathophysiology of schizophrenia, since, among other alterations, studies have described deficits in cortical PV interneurons, GABAergic dysfunction, and excitatory-inhibitory imbalance [69, 70].

PNNs have also been implicated in the pathophysiology of AD. In postmortem human brains, a significant loss of N-acetylgalactosamine residues, a key component of CSPGs in PNNs, has been observed in the frontal cortex of AD patients, suggesting PNN degradation [71]. Notably, this loss appears to be associated with fragmentation and disruption of the PNN structure without direct degeneration of the enwrapped PV interneurons [71]. In animal models, further evidence supports a detrimental impact of AD pathology on PNN integrity. In the 5xFAD mouse model of AD, a robust and age-dependent reduction in PNN number was detected, especially in brain regions with high amyloid-beta (A β) plaque burden, one of the key pathological hallmarks of the disease [4]. This observation suggests an inverse correlation between A β deposition and PNN expression. Moreover, supporting a possible neuroprotective role of PNNs, studies in human AD brains have shown that neurofibrillary tangles, another major hallmark of AD, are rarely found in regions rich in PNNs and neuropil-associated CSPGs. This observation points to a protective effect of CSPG-rich ECM structures against tau pathology [72, 73]. However, given that PNNs also restrict synaptic plasticity, their degradation may, paradoxically, offer transient functional and memory benefits. In mouse models of tauopathy, enzymatic digestion of PNNs in the perirhinal cortex using ch-ABC or masking specific sulfation patterns with antibodies against 4-sulfated chondroitin sulfate chains temporarily restored object recognition memory without affecting disease progression [74, 75]. These findings highlight the dualistic nature of PNN alterations in AD, where both their loss and persistence may influence disease outcomes in apparently opposing ways. This complex relationship between PNN integrity and AD pathogenesis underscores the importance of continued investigation into ECM dynamics as both a contributor to disease progression and a potential target for novel therapeutic strategies.

In the context of PD, PNNs have also emerged as critical regulators of cortical plasticity related to motor function. A recent study [6] revealed that transient degradation of PNNs in the primary motor cortex using ch-ABC in otherwise healthy adult mice leads to temporary motor deficits, indicating that PNNs contribute to the maintenance of normal motor function. In a unilateral 6-hydroxydopamine mouse model of PD, PNN levels were transiently reduced bilaterally in the primary motor cortex two weeks after the lesion but returned to baseline within five weeks [6]. Interestingly, a second transient PNN degradation in the motor cortex, when combined with motor training, was able to promote motor recovery. This functional improvement was accompanied by a bilateral increase in PNN-enwrapped PV interneurons and a rebalancing of excitatory synaptic markers on their somata [6]. These findings suggest a dual role for PNN plasticity: first, as a response to dopaminergic injury, and later, as a facilitator of functional recovery when paired with rehabilitation. Thus, PNNs in the motor cortex may represent promising therapeutic targets for enhancing motor rehabilitation in PD.

Growing evidence also links PNN abnormalities to ASD. A significant reduction in the number of PV interneurons enwrapped by PNNs has been detected in the globus pallidus of human postmortem brains from individuals with ASD [8]. In contrast, increased PNN density has been reported in brain regions involved in social behavior and somatosensory processing in Engrailed2 knock-out mice, a murine model of ASD [76]. Similarly, in a double-hit mouse model that combines maternal immune activation and hypoxia-ischemia, which induces ASD-like behaviors, researchers observed an enhanced infiltration of Otx2-expressing monocytes and an increase in PNN-surrounded PV neurons [77]. Interestingly, blocking monocyte infiltration led to a reduction in both autistic-like behaviors and the number of PNN-enwrapped PV cells [77]. In another study using the valproic acid mouse model of ASD, alterations in the PV-PNN relationship were detected in the prelimbic PFC [9]. Specifically, a decrease in PV expression alongside an increase in PNN intensity was reported. Remarkably, these abnormalities were normalized following ch-ABC treatment, suggesting the presence of a subpopulation of neurons with an altered PV/PNN ratio that may contribute to ASD-related pathology [9].

Alterations in PNN integrity have also been reported in models of epilepsy. In transgenic mouse models of the disease, PNN degradation by proteolytic enzymes has been described long before the onset of seizures and has been associated with the loss of PV interneurons and impaired presynaptic inhibition, both of which contribute to network hyperexcitability [10]. A decrease in PNN-enwrapped PV neurons has also been reported after the induction of experimental epilepsy. Notably, treatment with doxycycline, an inhibitor of MMPs, prevents PNN breakdown and the onset of seizures, suggesting that PNN degradation may be necessary for seizure development [78]. Supporting this view, enzymatic disruption of PNNs has been shown to exacerbate seizure susceptibility in response to pentylenetetrazole, leading to an increased number of myoclonic seizures [79].

Thus, studies conducted in both human brains and animal models highlight how alterations in PNN dynamics underscore their critical role in maintaining brain homeostasis and contribute to the development of neurological disorders. Understanding which cell types are capable of modulating the structure and function of PNNs is, therefore, essential, as these cells may represent promising targets for novel pharmacological interventions aimed at restoring neural plasticity or halting disease progression.

4. Microglia

Microglial cells were initially identified in 1919 by Pío del Río-Hortega, who named them and also described their distribution, morphological phenotype, and phagocytic capacity [80]. It was later discovered that these cells are part of the innate immune system and respond to pathogens and neuronal degeneration to protect and repair the brain, thereby maintaining its homeostasis. In recent decades, research on microglia has grown significantly and is currently a major focus within the neuroscience field.

As the resident macrophages of the CNS, microglia have highly motile processes that allow them to move through the brain parenchyma and continuously survey their environment, detecting changes and responding to them [81], which confers on them a vital role in brain physiology and disease as the housekeepers of the brain.

Microglia are the only brain-resident cells with a myeloid origin. They predominantly originate from yolk sac-derived macrophages during early embryogenesis and colonize the brain before neurons, other glial cells, and established vasculature, first appearing in the mouse brain around E9.5 [82, 83]. They then proliferate to eventually represent around 7% of non-neuronal brain cells [84], although their abundance depends on the brain region. Once the blood-brain barrier is formed, microglia are maintained by self-renewal, in a balance between proliferation and apoptosis [85]. To this end, microglial viability and proliferation are highly dependent on the colony-stimulating factor 1 receptor (CSF1R) signaling, and CSF1R inhibitors result in microglial depletion in the mouse brain [86].

Microglial homeostatic signature is characterized by the expression of certain genes, including P2RY12, Cx3cr1, and Tmem119 [87]. Nevertheless, heterogeneity is one of the characteristics of microglial cells, as even in homeostatic conditions, they can display diverse morphology, gene expression profiles, and functionality, depending not only on factors like age, sex, and other contextual cues but also in response to their microenvironment [88].

Microglia play a pivotal role in the immune response of the brain. They have toll-like receptors that recognize damage- and pathogen-associated molecular patterns. Upon activation of these receptors, microglia release cytokines (e.g., IL-1β, TNF-α, IL-6, IL-10, and TGF-β), and chemokines, transitioning to a reactive state characterized by ameboid morphology and increased phagocytic activity. They are able to engulf and digest pathogens, apoptotic cells, and cellular debris. This "reactive" state of microglia is common in many diseases and alterations and is referred to as damage-associated microglia (DAM) [88]. Although DAM microglia have been proposed to exert an initially protective role in response to harmful stimuli or adverse conditions, excessive or sustained microglial activation or microgliosis becomes detrimental. Microglia are not merely passive observers or secondary responders during disease but rather active players and modulators of the progression of brain pathology [89]. Indeed, such dysregulated microglial activity has been implicated in the pathogenesis of neurodegenerative and CNS diseases, including AD, multiple sclerosis, brain tumors, traumatic injury, and infection [90–95].

Microglia are also crucial to ensure the proper development of the CNS. They eliminate excess synaptic connections that form during the developmental period in a process known as synaptic pruning [96–98]. This is necessary for circuit refinement and the establishment of relevant neuronal connections.

Importantly, microglial function is essential for correct neuronal function. In fact, these cells can sense neuronal activity and respond to it. They are involved in circuit remodeling since they modulate synapses and dendritic spines and impact neuronal plasticity [99–101]. Beyond engulfing synaptic components, Eyo and Molofsky [102] propose additional mechanisms for microglia-synapse interactions. These include the engulfment of dying neurons and cell fragments for debris clearance, partial phagocytosis, or trogocytosis modifying the synapse without completely eliminating it, and physical interposition between pre- and post-synaptic elements, potentially limiting synaptic transmission. They also propose that microglia may remove ECM, thereby destabilizing synapses and contributing to synapse elimination [102]. Collectively, these mechanisms broaden the possibilities of microglia remodeling synapses beyond the traditional vision centered on engulfment and phagocytosis.

5. Microglia regulate perineuronal nets

In addition to their well-established roles in maintaining brain homeostasis in both health and disease, microglia also contribute to the regulation of PNN dynamics through multiple mechanisms (**Figure 2A**). Microglia act as key modulators of PNNs, in part by phagocytosing these ECM structures. This function is supported by studies demonstrating the presence of PNN components within microglia and their lysosomes in both human and mouse brains [4, 103]. Further evidence comes from experiments in animals where microglia are depleted using a CSF1R inhibitor. This treatment robustly decreases microglial cell numbers and results in a substantial increase in PNN density throughout the brain [104–106] (**Figure 2B**). Complementing these findings, other studies have shown that microglial modulation also affects the fine architecture of the ECM, even when overall PNN number or intensity remains unchanged. For instance, in the CA1 region of the hippocampus, microglial depletion leads to a reduction in PNN hole size and an increase in surrounding ECM components and perisynaptic brevican levels [107, 108]. These structural changes are accompanied by an increased number of Vglut1-positive presynaptic puncta, enhanced long-term potentiation, and improved performance in the hippocampus-dependent novel object location recognition task, suggesting that microglial regulation of PNNs has functional consequences on synaptic plasticity and cognition [107, 108].

Beyond phagocytosis, microglia also regulate PNNs through enzymatic degradation (**Figure 2A**). They express various proteolytic enzymes capable of breaking down PNN components, including MMP-2, MMP-9, ADAMTS-4, and cathepsins [109–111]. In a mouse model of amyotrophic lateral sclerosis, an increase in MMP-9 expressing microglia was observed, along with degradation of PNNs around α -motor neurons [112].

The mechanisms by which microglia interact with PNNs and modulate their structure and function remain largely unclear. However, several signaling molecules, such as interleukin-33 (IL-33), fractalkine (CX3CL1), and the purinergic receptor P2Y12, have emerged as potential mediators of this process (**Figure 2A**). IL-33 may promote microglial degradation of PNNs, since activation of its receptor on microglia induces the engulfment of the ECM by these cells [113]. This modification of the ECM promotes experience-dependent synaptic remodeling in the hippocampus, whereas IL-33 deficiency leads to ECM accumulation at synapses, decreased spine plasticity, and impaired memory consolidation [113].

Fractalkine signaling through its receptor CX3CR1 also seems to be critical for microglial modulation of PNNs. In the dorsal horn of the spinal cord, PNNs enwrap spinoparabrachial projection neurons involved in transmitting nociceptive signals to the brain. Tansley et al. [103] showed that microglial activation leads to PNN degradation around these neurons, increasing their excitability and resulting in pain hypersensitivity, findings consistent with previous reports by [114]. Notably, both microglial depletion and CX3CR1 knockout prevented PNN degradation and the associated pain response, suggesting that CX3CR1 signaling is required for microglia-mediated PNN remodeling in this context [103].

Similarly, Venturino et al. [115] found that microglial depletion prevented PNN loss induced by ketamine or 60-Hz light entrainment. Disruption of P2Y12 signaling, a key pathway through which microglia detect neuronal activity, produced the same protective effect against PNN loss [115]. These findings support the idea that microglial removal of PNNs is an activity-dependent process, with P2Y12 signaling playing a necessary role in mediating the microglial response to neuronal cues.

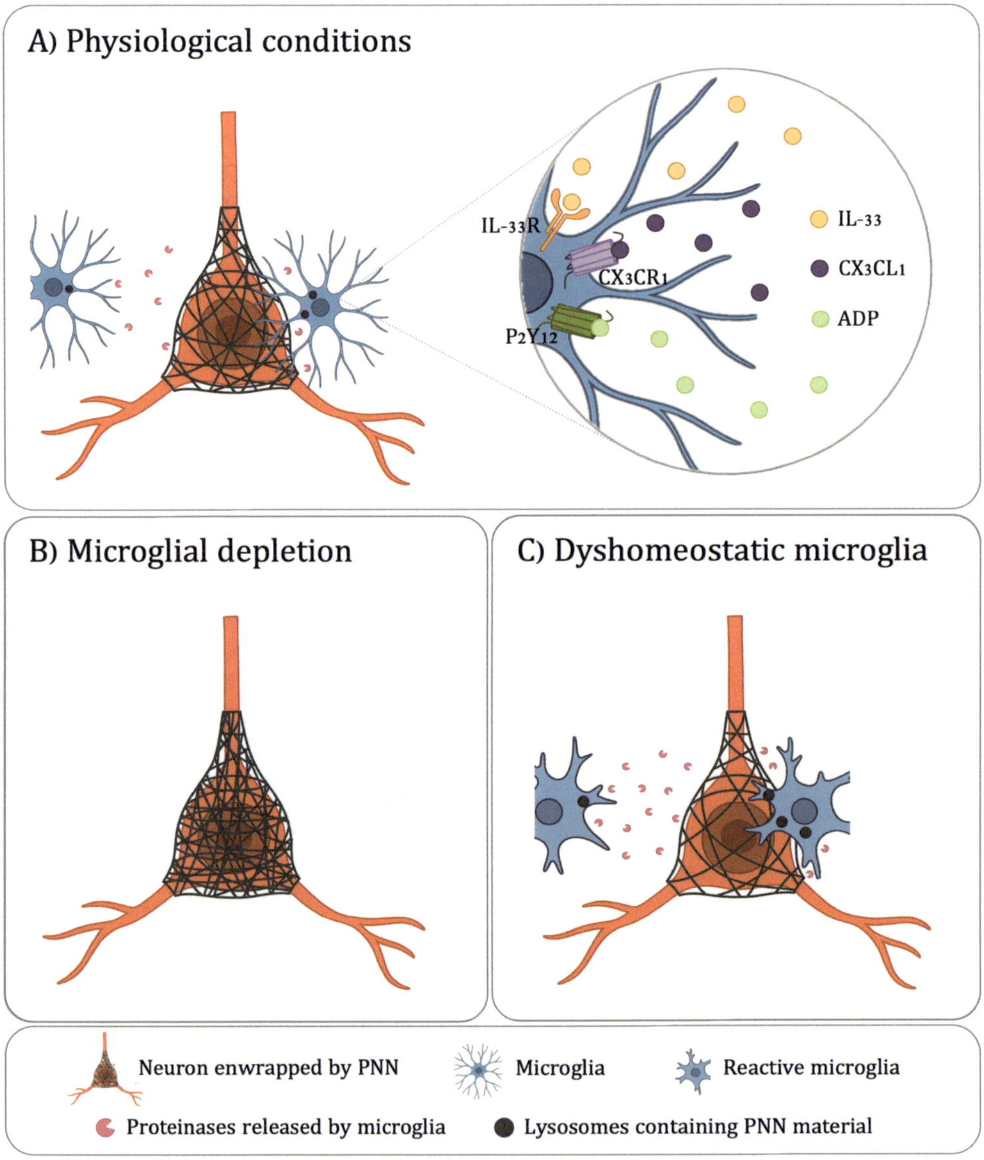

Figure 2.
Microglia regulate perineuronal nets (PNNs). (A) In physiological conditions, microglia phagocytose PNN components and release proteinases that digest PNNs. Some of the mechanisms triggering the degradation of PNNs by microglia might be the activation of receptors IL-33R, CX3CR1, and P2Y12. (B) Microglial depletion results in an increased density of PNNs. (C) Dyshomeostatic microglia are associated with an increase in the release of proteinases and phagocytic activity, resulting in dysfunctional PNNs.

5.1. Microglia regulate PNNs during development

Microglia play a pivotal role in shaping the structure and function of neural circuits during postnatal development, and emerging evidence indicates that their interactions with PNNs are central to this process. As mentioned above, PNNs emerge around the time that experience-dependent CPs end, suggesting a tight relationship between PNN formation and the timing of developmental plasticity. Microglia proliferate rapidly during the early postnatal period, with their numbers peaking around the third postnatal week and declining by 50% by the sixth week, aligning temporally with the progression of CP in regions such as the visual cortex [106]. Indeed, several studies have demonstrated that microglia are essential for visual cortex plasticity during the CP [106, 116]. In this scenario, a recent study has demonstrated that microglial elimination during this window increased PV expression and PNN density, while microglial repopulation reduced the number of PV interneurons and associated PNNs [106]. This dynamic regulation was shown to be functionally relevant: microglial depletion impaired ocular dominance plasticity, an effect that could be reversed upon treatment withdrawal. Additionally, alterations in miniature excitatory and inhibitory postsynaptic currents (mEPSCs and mIPSCs) in the primary visual cortex (V1) were observed, reflecting disrupted synaptic function and experience-dependent plasticity. Notably, the effects of microglial depletion were more pronounced on inhibitory neurons than on glutamatergic excitatory neurons [106]. These findings highlight a critical role for microglia in regulating the maturation of PV interneurons and the timing of CP closure via modulation of PNN deposition.

The importance of microglial regulation of PNNs during development extends beyond the visual cortex. A recent study by Sun et al. [117] explored this phenomenon in the hypothalamic arcuate nucleus (ARC), a region essential for metabolic regulation. The authors showed that microglial depletion during a postnatal critical window led to an increased number of Agouti-related peptide (AgRP) neurons and enhanced axonal fiber density, with comparatively minor effects on proopiomelanocortin (POMC) neurons. This was accompanied by increased neonatal feeding behavior, indicating a functional impact on metabolic circuits. Mechanistically, microglia was shown to engulf PNN components surrounding AgRP neurons both *in vivo* and *ex vivo*. Microglial depletion resulted in excessive PNN formation and heightened leptin sensitivity in the ARC, suggesting that microglia actively regulate PNN remodeling to shape hypothalamic neuron maturation and energy balance [117].

Together, these findings underscore the essential contribution of microglia to the regulation of PNNs across different brain regions during development. By controlling the timing and extent of PNN deposition, microglia influence neuronal maturation, circuit connectivity, and the closure of CPs of plasticity. These insights not only reveal a previously underappreciated aspect of microglial function but also open new avenues for understanding how disruptions in microglia-PNN interactions during development may contribute to neurodevelopmental and metabolic disorders.

5.2. Dyshomeostatic microglia disrupt PNN in pathological conditions

Since correct microglial function is essential for maintaining the structural and functional integrity of PNNs, it is not surprising that microglial activation under pathological conditions can disrupt PNN structure (**Figure 2C**), with significant consequences for neuronal function. In vitro studies have shown that microglial activation with Poly I:C increases the release of proinflammatory cytokines and MMPs. Conditioned media from these activated microglia was able to disrupt PNNs of cultured hippocampal neurons, resulting in altered synaptic plasticity and electrophysiological properties [118]. Similarly, in ME7 murine model of prion disease, characterized by early microglial activation, PNN degradation has been attributed to reactive microglia. This degradation is accompanied by synaptic dysfunction and behavioral deficits, suggesting that microglial-mediated PNN disruption contributes to the early pathological changes observed in this model [119]. Further supporting this concept, microglial depletion in both AD and Huntington's disease mouse models prevents PNN loss, suggesting that activated microglia are responsible for the PNN disruption in neurodegenerative contexts [4, 105]. In line with these findings, microglial dyshomeostasis caused by the specific reduction of CSF1R in adult microglia was sufficient to induce PNN degradation and loss of presynaptic markers [120]. Beyond animal models, recent evidence supports a role for microglia in modulating PNNs in the human brain as well. A recent study by Belliveau et al. [121] analyzed postmortem samples from individuals with a history of childhood abuse and reported increased PNN density in the ventromedial prefrontal cortex (vmPFC), consistent with earlier findings [122]. This increase was accompanied by reduced expression of microglial receptors IL-33 R and CX3CR1 as well as lower levels of MMP-9 and its regulator TIMP-2, both in the whole gray matter of the vmPFC and isolated microglia [121]. These results suggest that microglial dysfunction may contribute to PNN alterations in humans, potentially linking early-life adversity to long-term changes in ECM and neuronal plasticity.

Taken together, these findings highlight microglia as central regulators of PNN homeostasis throughout life, including both developmental and pathological contexts. Their dysregulation contributes to PNN disruption and associated neuronal dysfunction across a wide range of brain disorders. Therefore, continued investigation into microglia–PNN interactions in a context- and disease-specific manner holds great promise for the identification of novel therapeutic strategies. Modulating microglial activity to restore ECM balance and PNN integrity may represent a promising approach to preserving or recovering neuronal function in both neurological and psychiatric conditions.

6. Conclusions

PNNs are dynamic structures that extensively influence neuronal function and synaptic plasticity. They play a crucial role in ensuring the proper closure of CPs during neurodevelopment and limiting plasticity thereafter, while also having a neuroprotective effect. Their relevance goes beyond a physiological role, as alterations in their structure and functionality are present in major neurological diseases and disorders such as schizophrenia, AD, and ASD. The need for new therapeutic approaches to target these conditions positions the modulation of PNNs as a potential objective and topic of study. In this context, regulation of microglial function could be a prospective candidate, given that these cells highly influence the densities and integrity of PNNs in both physiological and pathological conditions. Nevertheless, in order to put forward any approach that includes PNN modulation via microglial manipulation, extensive research is required in the field of microglial interactions with PNNs and the mechanisms involved.

Acknowledgments

This work was supported by grant PID2020-119729GB-I00, funded by MICIU/AEI/10.13039/501100011033, to E.P. We also gratefully acknowledge the support of "Amigos de la Universidad de Navarra" and the Spanish Ministry of Universities for a fellowship awarded to M.G.-B.

Conflict of interest

The authors declare no conflicts of interest.

Author details

Maider Garmendia-Berges and Elena Puerta*

1 Department of Pharmaceutical Sciences, University of Navarra, Pamplona, Spain

2 Navarra Institute for Health Research (IdiSNA), Pamplona, Spain

*Address all correspondence to: epuerta@unav.es

References

[1] Syková E, Nicholson C.Diffusion in brain extracellular space. Physiological Reviews. 2008;**88**(4):1277–1340

[2] Dityatev A, Rusakov DA.Molecular signals of plasticity at the tetrapartite synapse. Current Opinion in Neurobiology. 2011;**21**(2):353–359

[3] Crapser JD, Arreola MA, Tsourmas KI, Green KN.Microglia as hackers of the matrix: Sculpting synapses and the extracellular space. Cellular and Molecular Immunology. 2021;**18** (11):2472–2488

[4] Crapser JD, Spangenberg EE, Barahona RA, Arreola MA, Hohsfield LA, Green KN. Microglia facilitate loss of perineuronal nets in the Alzheimer's disease brain. EBioMedicine. 2020;**58**:102919. 102919.

[5] Logsdon AF, Foresi B, Hu SJ, Quah E, Meuret CJ, Le JP, et al. Perineuronal net deglycosylation associates with tauopathy-induced gliosis and neurodegeneration. Journal of Neurochemistry 2024;**168**:1923–1936

[6] Benacom D, Chataing C, Prochiantz A, Di Nardo AA. Motor recovery through perineuronal net modulation in a Parkinson's disease mouse model. Brain. 2025;awaf226

[7] Garcia-Mompo C, Curto Y, Carceller H, Gilabert-Juan J, Rodriguez-Flores E, Guirado R, et al. Δ-9-Tetrahydrocannabinol treatment during adolescence and alterations in the inhibitory networks of the adult prefrontal cortex in mice subjected to perinatal NMDA receptor antagonist injection and to postweaning social isolation. Translational Psychiatry 2020;**10**:177

[8] Brandenburg C, Blatt GJ. Region-specific alterations of perineuronal net expression in postmortem autism Brain tissue. Frontiers in Molecular Neuroscience. 2022;**15**:838918.

[9] Xia D, Li L, Yang B, Zhou Q. Altered relationship between parvalbumin and perineuronal nets in an Autism model. Frontiers in Molecular Neuroscience. 2021;**14**:597812.

[10] Yang T, Hu S, Chang WC, Kao HY, Wang Y.Perineuronal nets degradation and parvalbumin interneuron loss in a mouse model of DEPDC5-related epilepsy. Developmental Neuroscience. 2022;**44**(6):671–677

[11] Zhu K, Fu Y, Zhao Y, Niu B, Lu H. Perineuronal nets: Role in normal brain physiology and aging, and pathology of various diseases. Ageing Research Reviews. 2025;**108**:102756.

[12] Auer S, Schicht M, Hoffmann L, Budday S, Frischknecht R, Blümcke I, et al. The role of perineuronal nets in physiology and disease: insights from recent studies. Cells 2025;**14**:321

[13] Beurdeley M, Spatazza J, Lee HHC, Sugiyama S, Bernard C, Di Nardo AA, et al. Otx2 binding to perineuronal nets persistently regulates plasticity in the mature visual cortex. Journal of Neuroscience 2012;**32**:9429–9437

[14] Boggio EM, EM E, Lupori L, EB M, De Winter F, Vander Kooi CW, et al. Inhibition of Semaphorin3A promotes ocular dominance plasticity in the adult

rat visual cortex. Molecular Neurobiology 2019;**56**:5987–5997

[15] Van't Spijker HM, Rowlands D, Rossier J, Haenzi B, Fawcett JW, Kwok JCF. Neuronal pentraxin 2 binds PNNs and enhances PNN formation. Neural Plasticity. 2019;**2019**:1–13. 6804575.

[16] Fawcett JW, Fyhn M, Jendelova P, Kwok JCF, Ruzicka J, Sorg BA.The extracellular matrix and perineuronal nets in memory. Molecular Psychiatry. 2022;**27**(8):3192–3203

[17] Soles A, Selimovic A, Sbrocco K, Ghannoum F, Hamel K, Moncada EL, et al. Extracellular matrix regulation in physiology and in brain disease. International Journal of Molecular Sciences 2023;**24**:7049

[18] Celio MR.Perineuronal nets of extracellular matrix around parvalbumin-containing neurons of the hippocampus. Hippocampus. 1993;**3** (S1):55–60

[19] Kosaka T, Heizmann CW, Barnstable CJ.Monoclonal antibody VC1.1 selectively stains a population of GABAergic neurons containing the calcium-binding protein parvalbumin in the rat cerebral cortex. Experimental Brain Research. 1989;**78**(1):43–50

[20] Härtig W, Brauer K, Brückner G. Wisteria floribunda agglutinin-labelled nets surround parvalbumin-containing neurons. Neuroreport. 1992;**3**(10):869–872

[21] Wegner F, Härtig W, Bringmann A, Grosche J, Wohlfarth K, Zuschratter W, et al. Diffuse perineuronal nets and modified pyramidal cells immunoreactive for glutamate and the GABA(A) receptor alpha1 subunit form a unique entity in rat cerebral cortex. Experimental Neurology 2003;**184**:705–714

[22] Morikawa S, Ikegaya Y, Narita M, Tamura H. Activation of perineuronal net-expressing excitatory neurons during associative memory encoding and retrieval. Scientific Reports. 2017;**7**:46024.

[23] Vitellaro-Zuccarello L, Bosisio P, Mazzetti S, Monti C, De Biasi S. Differential expression of several molecules of the extracellular matrix in functionally and developmentally distinct regions of rat spinal cord. Cell and Tissue Research. 2007;**327**(3):433–447

[24] Alpár A, Gärtner U, Härtig W, Brückner G.Distribution of pyramidal cells associated with perineuronal nets in the neocortex of rat. Brain Research. 2006;**1120**(1):13–22

[25] Carstens KE, Phillips ML, Pozzo-Miller L, Weinberg RJ, Dudek SM. Perineuronal nets suppress plasticity of excitatory synapses on CA2 pyramidal neurons. The Journal of Neuroscience. 2016;**36**(23):6312–6320

[26] Sahin M, Hockfield S.Molecular identification of the lugaro cell in the cat cerebellar cortex. Journal of Comparative Neurology. 1990;**301** (4):575–584

[27] Corvetti L, Rossi F.Degradation of chondroitin sulfate proteoglycans induces sprouting of intact purkinje axons in the cerebellum of the adult rat. The Journal of Neuroscience. 2005;**25** (31):7150–7158

[28] Carulli D, Broersen R, de Winter F, Muir EM, Mešković M, de Waal M, et al. Cerebellar plasticity and associative memories are controlled by

perineuronal nets. Proceedings of the National Academy of Sciences 2020;**117**:6855–6865

[29] Kind PC, Sengpiel F, Beaver CJ, Crocker-Buque A, Kelly GM, Matthews RT, et al. The development and activity-dependent expression of aggrecan in the cat visual cortex. Cerebral Cortex 2013;**23**:349–360

[30] Myers AK, Ray J, Kulesza RJ. Neonatal conductive hearing loss disrupts the development of the Cat-315 epitope on perineuronal nets in the rat superior olivary complex. Brain Research. 2012;**1465**:34–47

[31] McRae PA, Rocco MM, Kelly G, Brumberg JC, Matthews RT.Sensory deprivation alters aggrecan and perineuronal net expression in the mouse barrel cortex. The Journal of Neuroscience. 2007;**27**(20):5405–5413

[32] Fawcett JW, Oohashi T, Pizzorusso T.The roles of perineuronal nets and the perinodal extracellular matrix in neuronal function. Nature Reviews, Neuroscience. 2019;**20**(8):451–465

[33] Carulli D, Pizzorusso T, Kwok JCF, Putignano E, Poli A, Forostyak S, et al. Animals lacking link protein have attenuated perineuronal nets and persistent plasticity. Brain 2010;**133**:2331–2347

[34] Pizzorusso T, Medini P, Berardi N, Chierzi S, Fawcett JW, Maffei L. Reactivation of ocular dominance plasticity in the adult visual cortex. Science. 2002;**298**(5596):1248–1251

[35] Pizzorusso T, Medini P, Landi S, Baldini S, Berardi N, Maffei L.Structural and functional recovery from early monocular deprivation in adult rats. Proceedings of the National Academy of Sciences. 2006;**103**(22):8517–8522

[36] Lensjø KK, Lepperød ME, Dick G, Hafting T, Fyhn M.Removal of perineuronal nets unlocks Juvenile plasticity through network mechanisms of decreased inhibition and increased Gamma activity. The Journal of Neuroscience. 2017;**37**(5):1269–1283

[37] Sugiyama S, Di Nardo AA, Aizawa S, Matsuo I, Volovitch M, Prochiantz A, et al. Experience-dependent transfer of Otx2 homeoprotein into the visual cortex activates postnatal plasticity. Cell 2008;**134**:508–520

[38] Lee HHC, Bernard C, Ye Z, Acampora D, Simeone A, Prochiantz A, et al. Genetic Otx2 mis-localization delays critical period plasticity across brain regions. Molecular Psychiatry 2017;**22**:680–688

[39] Spatazza J, Lee HHC, Di Nardo AA, Tibaldi L, Joliot A, Hensch TK, et al. Choroid-plexus-derived Otx2 homeoprotein constrains adult cortical plasticity. Cell Reports 2013;**3**:1815–1823

[40] Miyata S, Komatsu Y, Yoshimura Y, Taya C, Kitagawa H.Persistent cortical plasticity by upregulation of chondroitin 6-sulfation. Nature Neuroscience. 2012;**15**(3):414–22,S1–2

[41] Lin R, Rosahl TW, Whiting PJ, Fawcett JW, Kwok JCF. 6-Sulphated chondroitins have a positive influence on axonal regeneration. PLoS One. 2011;**6**(7)

[42] Wang H, Katagiri Y, McCann TE, Unsworth E, Goldsmith P, Yu ZX, et al. Chondroitin-4-sulfation negatively

regulates axonal guidance and growth. Journal of Cell Science 2008;**121**: 3083–3091

[43] Wang D, Fawcett J.The perineuronal net and the control of CNS plasticity. Cell and Tissue Research. 2012;**349**(1):147–160

[44] Sorg BA, Berretta S, Blacktop JM, Fawcett JW, Kitagawa H, Kwok JCF, et al. Casting a wide net: Role of Perineuronal nets in neural plasticity. The Journal of Neuroscience 2016;**36**:11459–11468

[45] Barritt AW, Davies M, Marchand F, Hartley R, Grist J, Yip P, et al. Chondroitinase ABC promotes sprouting of intact and injured spinal systems after spinal cord injury. The Journal of Neuroscience 2006;**26**: 10856–10867

[46] Wang D, Ichiyama RM, Zhao R, Andrews MR, Fawcett JW. Chondroitinase combined with rehabilitation promotes recovery of forelimb function in rats with chronic spinal cord injury. Journal of Neuroscience. 2011;**31**(25): 9332–9344

[47] Deepa SS, Umehara Y, Higashiyama S, Itoh N, Sugahara K. Specific molecular interactions of oversulfated chondroitin sulfate E with various heparin-binding growth factors. Implications as a physiological binding partner in the brain and other tissues. Journal of Biological Chemistry. 2002;**277**(46): 43707–43716

[48] Frischknecht R, Heine M, Perrais D, Seidenbecher CI, Choquet D, Gundelfinger ED.Brain extracellular matrix affects AMPA receptor lateral mobility and short-term synaptic plasticity. Nature Neuroscience. 2009;**12**(7):897–904

[49] Hylin MJ, Orsi SA, Moore AN, Dash PK.Disruption of the perineuronal net in the hippocampus or medial prefrontal cortex impairs fear conditioning. Learning & Memory. 2013;**20**(5):267–273

[50] Gogolla N, Caroni P, Lüthi A, Herry C.Perineuronal nets protect fear memories from erasure. Science. 2009;**325**(5945):1258–1261

[51] Alexander GM, Nikolova VD, Stöber TM, Gruzdev A, Moy SS, Dudek SM.Perineuronal nets on CA2 pyramidal cells and parvalbumin-expressing cells differentially regulate hippocampal-dependent memory. The Journal of Neuroscience. 2025;**45**(6): e1626242024

[52] Huang H, Joffrin AM, Zhao Y, Miller GM, Zhang GC, Oka Y, et al. Chondroitin 4-O-sulfation regulates hippocampal perineuronal nets and social memory. Proceedings of the National Academy of Sciences USA 2023;**120**:e2301312120

[53] Rowlands D, Lensjø KK, Dinh T, Yang S, Andrews MR, Hafting T, et al. Aggrecan directs extracellular matrix-mediated neuronal plasticity. The Journal of Neuroscience 2018;**38**:10102–10113

[54] Romberg C, Yang S, Melani R, Andrews MR, Horner AE, Spillantini MG, et al. Depletion of perineuronal nets enhances recognition memory and long-term depression in the perirhinal cortex. The Journal of Neuroscience 2013;**33**:7057–7065

[55] Brückner G, Brauer K, Härtig W, Wolff JR, Rickmann MJ, Derouiche A, et

al. Perineuronal nets provide a polyanionic, Glia-associated form of microenvironment around certain neurons in many parts of the rat brain. Glia 1993;**8**:183–200

[56] Morawski M, Reinert T, Meyer-Klaucke W, Wagner FE, Tröger W, Reinert A, et al. Ion exchanger in the brain: Quantitative analysis of perineuronally fixed anionic binding sites suggests diffusion barriers with ion sorting properties. Scientific Reports. 2015;**5**:16471.

[57] Härtig W, Derouiche A, Welt K, Brauer K, Grosche J, Mäder M, et al. Cortical neurons immunoreactive for the potassium channel Kv3.1b subunit are predominantly surrounded by perineuronal nets presumed as a buffering system for cations. Brain Research 1999;**842**:15–29

[58] Hrabětová S, Masri D, Tao L, Xiao F, Nicholson C.Calcium diffusion enhanced after cleavage of negatively charged components of brain extracellular matrix by chondroitinase ABC. The Journal of Physiology. 2009;**587**(16):4029–4049

[59] Balmer TS. Perineuronal nets enhance the excitability of fast-spiking neurons. eNeuro. 2016; ENEURO.0112-16.2016 **3**(4): ENEURO.0112–16.2016.

[60] Morawski M, Brückner MK, Riederer P, Brückner G, Arendt T. Perineuronal nets potentially protect against oxidative stress. Experimental Neurology. 2004;**188**(2):309–315

[61] Suttkus A, Rohn S, Jäger C, Arendt T, Morawski M.Neuroprotection against iron-induced cell death by perineuronal nets - an in vivo analysis of oxidative stress. American Journal of Neurodegenerative Disease. 2012;**1**(2):122–129

[62] Suttkus A, Rohn S, Weigel S, Glöckner P, Arendt T, Morawski M. Aggrecan, link protein and tenascin-R are essential components of the perineuronal net to protect neurons against iron-induced oxidative stress. Cell Death and Disease. 2014;**5**(3):e1119

[63] Cabungcal JH, Steullet P, Morishita H, Kraftsik R, Cuenod M, Hensch TK, et al. Perineuronal nets protect fast-spiking interneurons against oxidative stress. Proceedings of the National Academy of Sciences USA 2013;**110**:9130–9135

[64] Mauney SA, Athanas KM, Pantazopoulos H, Shaskan N, Passeri E, Berretta S, et al. Developmental pattern of perineuronal nets in the human prefrontal cortex and their deficit in schizophrenia. Biological Psychiatry 2013;**74**:427–435

[65] Pantazopoulos H, Woo TUW, Lim MP, Lange N, Berretta S.Extracellular matrix-glial abnormalities in the amygdala and entorhinal cortex of subjects diagnosed with schizophrenia. Archives of General Psychiatry. 2010;**67**(2):155–166

[66] Enwright JF, Sanapala S, Foglio A, Berry R, Fish KN, Lewis DA.Reduced labeling of Parvalbumin neurons and Perineuronal nets in the dorsolateral prefrontal cortex of subjects with Schizophrenia. Neuropsychopharmacology. 2016;**41**(9):2206–2214

[67] Matuszko G, Curreli S, Kaushik R, Becker A, Dityatev A. Extracellular matrix alterations in the ketamine model of schizophrenia. Neuroscience. 2017;**350**:13–22

[68] Cabungcal JH, Steullet P, Kraftsik R, Cuenod M, Do KQ. A developmental redox dysregulation leads to spatio-temporal deficit of parvalbumin neuron circuitry in a schizophrenia mouse model. Schizophrenia Research. 2019;**213**:96–106

[69] Liu Y, Ouyang P, Zheng Y, Mi L, Zhao J, Ning Y, et al. A selective review of the excitatory-inhibitory imbalance in schizophrenia: Underlying biology, genetics, microcircuits, and symptoms. Frontiers in Cell and Developmental Biology. 2021;**9**:664535.

[70] Marín O. Parvalbumin interneuron deficits in schizophrenia. European Neuropsychopharmacology. 2024;**82**:44–52

[71] Baig S, Wilcock GK, Love S.Loss of perineuronal net N-acetylgalactosamine in Alzheimer's disease. Acta Neuropathologica. 2005;**110**(4):393–401

[72] Brückner G, Hausen D, Härtig W, Drlicek M, Arendt T, Brauer K.Cortical areas abundant in extracellular matrix chondroitin sulphate proteoglycans are less affected by cytoskeletal changes in Alzheimer's disease. Neuroscience. 1999;**92**(3):791–805

[73] Morawski M, Brückner G, Jäger C, Seeger G, Arendt T.Neurons associated with aggrecan-based perineuronal nets are protected against tau pathology in subcortical regions in Alzheimer's disease. Neuroscience. 2010;**169**(3):1347–1363

[74] Yang S, Cacquevel M, Saksida LM, Bussey TJ, Schneider BL, Aebischer P, et al. Perineuronal net digestion with chondroitinase restores memory in mice with tau pathology. Experimental Neurology. 2015;**265**:48–58

[75] Yang S, Hilton S, Alves JN, Saksida LM, Bussey T, Matthews RT, et al. Antibody recognizing 4-sulfated chondroitin sulfate proteoglycans restores memory in tauopathy-induced neurodegeneration. Neurobiology of Aging. 2017;**59**:197–209

[76] Mattioni L, Barbieri A, Grigoli A, Balasco L, Bozzi Y, Provenzano G. Alterations of perineuronal net expression and abnormal social behavior and whisker-dependent texture discrimination in mice lacking the autism candidate gene engrailed 2. Neuroscience. 2024;**546**:63–74

[77] HR C, CW C, Mandhani N, Short-Miller JC, Smucker MR, Sun YY, et al. Monocytic infiltrates contribute to autistic-like behaviors in a two-hit model of neurodevelopmental defects. The Journal of Neuroscience 2020;**40**:9386–9400

[78] Pollock E, Everest M, Brown A, Poulter MO. Metalloproteinase inhibition prevents inhibitory synapse reorganization and seizure genesis. Neurobiology of Disease. 2014;**70**:21–31

[79] Rankin-Gee EK, McRae PA, Baranov E, Rogers S, Wandrey L, Porter BE.Perineuronal net degradation in epilepsy. Epilepsia. 2015;**56**(7):1124–1133

[80] Sierra A, de Castro F, Del Río-Hortega J, Rafael Iglesias-Rozas J, Garrosa M, Kettenmann H.The "Big-Bang" for modern glial biology: Translation and comments on Pío del Río-Hortega 1919 series of papers on microglia. Glia. 2016;**64**(11):1801–1840

[81] Nimmerjahn A, Kirchhoff F, Helmchen F.Resting microglial cells are highly dynamic surveillants of brain parenchyma in vivo. Science. 2005;**308**(5726):1314–1318

[82] Alliot F, Godin I, Pessac B. Microglia derive from progenitors, originating from the yolk sac, and which proliferate in the brain. Developmental Brain Research. 1999;**117**(2):145–152

[83] Ginhoux F, Greter M, Leboeuf M, Nandi S, See P, Gokhan S, et al. Fate mapping analysis reveals that adult microglia derive from primitive macrophages. Science 2010;**330**: 841–845

[84] Dos Santos SE, Medeiros M, Porfirio J, Tavares W, Pessôa L, Grinberg L, et al. Similar microglial cell densities across brain structures and mammalian species: Implications for brain tissue function. The Journal of Neuroscience 2020;**40**:4622–4643

[85] Askew K, Li K, Olmos-Alonso A, Garcia-Moreno F, Liang Y, Richardson P, et al. Coupled proliferation and apoptosis maintain the rapid turnover of Microglia in the adult brain. Cell Reports 2017;**18**:391–405

[86] Elmore MRP, Najafi AR, Koike MA, Dagher NN, Spangenberg EE, Rice RA, et al. Colony-stimulating factor 1 receptor signaling is necessary for microglia viability, unmasking a microglia progenitor cell in the adult brain. Neuron 2014;**82**:380–397

[87] Boche D, Gordon MN.Diversity of transcriptomic microglial phenotypes in aging and Alzheimer's disease. Alzheimer's & Dementia. 2022;**18** (2):360–376

[88] Paolicelli RC, Sierra A, Stevens B, Tremblay ME, Aguzzi A, Ajami B, et al. Microglia states and nomenclature: A field at its crossroads. Neuron 2022;**110**:3458–3483

[89] Sierra A, Miron VE, Paolicelli RC, Ransohoff RM.Microglia in health and diseases: Integrative hubs of the Central Nervous System (CNS). Cold Spring Harbor Perspectives in Biology. 2024;**16** (8):a041366

[90] Loane DJ, Kumar A.Microglia in the TBI brain: The good, the bad, and the dysregulated. Experimental Neurology. 2016;**275**(Pt 3(03)):316–327

[91] Masuda T, Sankowski R, Staszewski O, Böttcher C, Amann L, Null S, et al. Spatial and temporal heterogeneity of mouse and human microglia at single-cell resolution. Nature 2019;**566**:388–392

[92] Young AMH, Kumasaka N, Calvert F, Hammond TR, Knights A, Panousis N, et al. A map of transcriptional heterogeneity and regulatory variation in human microglia. Nature Genetics 2021;**53**:861–868

[93] Xu Y, Gao W, Sun Y, Wu M. New insight on microglia activation in neurodegenerative diseases and therapeutics. Frontiers in Neuroscience. 2023;**17**:1308345.

[94] Keane L, Cheray M, Blomgren K, Joseph B.Multifaceted microglia - key players in primary brain tumour heterogeneity. Nature Reviews Neurology. 2021;**17**(4):243–259

[95] Ismail FS, TJ F, PM F, Corvace F. Microglia as potential key regulators in viral-induced neuroinflammation. Frontiers in Cellular Neuroscience. 2024;**18**:1426079.

[96] Paolicelli RC, Bolasco G, Pagani F, Maggi L, Scianni M, Panzanelli P, et al. Synaptic pruning by microglia is

necessary for normal brain development. Science 2011;**333**:1456–1458

[97] Schafer DP, Lehrman EK, Stevens B.The "quad-partite" synapse: Microglia-synapse interactions in the developing and mature CNS. Glia. 2013;**61**(1):24–36

[98] Mordelt A, de Witte LD. Microglia-mediated synaptic pruning as a key deficit in neurodevelopmental disorders: Hype or hope? Current Opinion in Neurobiology. 2023;**79**:102674.

[99] Pfeiffer T, Avignone E, Nägerl UV. Induction of hippocampal long-term potentiation increases the morphological dynamics of microglial processes and prolongs their contacts with dendritic spines. Scientific Reports. 2016;**6**:32422.

[100] Parkhurst CN, Yang G, Ninan I, Savas JN, Yates JR, Lafaille JJ, et al. Microglia promote learning-dependent synapse formation through brain-derived neurotrophic factor. Cell 2013;**155**:1596–1609

[101] Cangalaya C, Stoyanov S, Fischer KD, Dityatev A. Light-induced engagement of microglia to focally remodel synapses in the adult brain. eLife. 2020;**9**:e58435

[102] Eyo U, Molofsky AV.Defining microglial-synapse interactions. Science. 2023;**381**(6663):1155–1156

[103] Tansley S, Gu N, Guzmán AU, Cai W, Wong C, Lister KC, et al. Microglia-mediated degradation of perineuronal nets promotes pain. Science 2022;**377**:80–86

[104] Liu YJ, Spangenberg EE, Tang B, Holmes TC, Green KN, Xu X.Microglia elimination increases neural circuit connectivity and activity in adult mouse cortex. The Journal of Neuroscience. 2021;**41**(6):1274–1287

[105] Crapser JD, Ochaba J, Soni N, Reidling JC, Thompson LM, Green KN. Microglial depletion prevents extracellular matrix changes and striatal volume reduction in a model of Huntington's disease. Brain. 2020;**143** (1):266–288

[106] Wang X, Li K, Guo L, Liu X, Guo Y, Zhang W.The influence of changes in Microglia development on the plasticity of the developing visual cortex circuit in Juvenile mice. Investigative Ophthalmology and Visual Science. 2025;**66**(4):45

[107] Strackeljan L, Baczynska E, Cangalaya C, Baidoe-Ansah D, Wlodarczyk J, Kaushik R, et al. Microglia Depletion-Induced Remodeling of Extracellular Matrix and Excitatory Synapses in the Hippocampus of Adult Mice. Cells 2021;**10**:1862

[108] Strackeljan L, Baidoe-Ansah D, Mirzapourdelavar H, Jia S, Kaushik R, Cangalaya C, et al. Partial microglial depletion through inhibition of colony-stimulating factor 1 receptor improves synaptic plasticity and cognitive performance in aged mice. Experimental Neurology. 2025;**387**:115186.

[109] Nakanishi H. Cathepsin regulation on microglial function. Biochimica Et Biophysica Acta (BBA) - Proteins and Proteomics. 2020;**1868** (9):140465.

[110] Lemarchant S, Pruvost M, Montaner J, Emery E, Vivien D, Kanninen K, et al. ADAMTS

proteoglycanases in the physiological and pathological central nervous system. Journal of Neuroinflammation. 2013;**10**:133

[111] Könnecke H, Bechmann I. The role of microglia and matrix metalloproteinases involvement in neuroinflammation and gliomas. Clinical & Developmental Immunology. 2013;**2013**:1–15. 914104.

[112] Cheung SW, Bhavnani E, Simmons DG, Bellingham MC, Noakes PG. Perineuronal nets are phagocytosed by MMP-9 expressing microglia and astrocytes in the SOD1 G93A ALS mouse model. Neuropathology and Applied Neurobiology. 2024;**50**(3):e12982

[113] Nguyen PT, Dorman LC, Pan S, Vainchtein ID, Han RT, Nakao-Inoue H, et al. Microglial remodeling of the extracellular matrix promotes Synapse plasticity. Cell 2020;**182**:388–403.e15

[114] Yi MH, Liu YU, Umpierre AD, Chen T, Ying Y, Zheng J, et al. Optogenetic activation of spinal microglia triggers chronic pain in mice. Emery B, editor. PLOS Biology 2021;**19**: e3001154

[115] Venturino A, Schulz R, De Jesús-Cortés H, Maes ME, Nagy B, Reilly-Andújar F, et al. Microglia enable mature perineuronal nets disassembly upon anesthetic ketamine exposure or 60-Hz light entrainment in the healthy brain. Cell Reports. 2021;**361**:109313.

[116] Sipe GO, Lowery RL, Mè T, Kelly EA, Lamantia CE, Majewska AK. Microglial P2Y12 is necessary for synaptic plasticity in mouse visual cortex. Nature Communications. 2016;7:10905.

[117] Sun J, Wang X, Sun R, Xiao X, Wang Y, Peng Y, et al. Microglia shape AgRP neuron postnatal development via regulating perineuronal net plasticity. Molecular Psychiatry 2024;**29**:306–316

[118] Wegrzyn D, Freund N, Faissner A, Juckel G. Poly I:C activated microglia disrupt perineuronal nets and modulate synaptic balance in primary hippocampal neurons in vitro. Frontiers in Synaptic Neuroscience. 2021;**13**:637549.

[119] Franklin SL, Love S, Greene JRT, Betmouni S.Loss of Perineuronal Net in ME7 Prion Disease. Journal of Neuropathology and Experimental Neurology. 2008;**67**(3):189–199

[120] Arreola MA, Soni N, Crapser JD, Hohsfield LA, Elmore MRP, Matheos DP, et al. Microglial dyshomeostasis drives perineuronal net and synaptic loss in a CSF1R+/– mouse model of ALSP, which can be rescued via CSF1R inhibitors. Science Advances 2021;7: eabg1601

[121] Belliveau C, Rahimian R, Fakhfouri G, Hosdey C, Simard S, Davoli MA, et al. Evidence of microglial involvement in the childhood abuse-associated increase in perineuronal nets in the ventromedial prefrontal cortex. Brain, Behavior, and Immunity. 2025;**124**:321–334

[122] Tanti A, Belliveau C, Nagy C, Maitra M, Denux F, Perlman K, et al. Child abuse associates with increased recruitment of perineuronal nets in the ventromedial prefrontal cortex: A possible implication of oligodendrocyte progenitor cells. Molecular Psychiatry 2022;**27**:1552–1561

Section 3

Myelin Formation and Plasticity

Chapter 3

Myelin Formation and Plasticity in the Central Nervous System

Julie Pilon and Lamia Bouslama-Oueghlani

Abstract

During development, oligodendrocytes generate myelin sheaths that insulate axons, thereby enabling rapid signal conduction and providing essential metabolic support to neurons in the central nervous system (CNS). Subsequent to its initial formation, myelin undergoes adaptive remodeling in response to neuronal activity and environmental stimuli, thereby enabling dynamic regulation of neuronal circuits throughout life. Myelin formation and plasticity are critical for efficient neuronal communication, and disruptions in these processes have been implicated in neurodegenerative diseases and psychiatric disorders such as multiple sclerosis, leukodystrophies, and autism spectrum disorders. Therefore, elucidating the molecular mechanisms that govern myelin dynamics is essential for the development of strategies to preserve or restore CNS function. This chapter provides a comprehensive overview of the structural complexity of myelin, elucidates some of the molecular mechanisms that underpin its formation, and underscores its adaptive characteristics, particularly myelin plasticity in behavior.

Keywords: myelin, oligodendrocytes, OPCs, development, plasticity, behavior

1. Introduction

Myelin is a multilamellar stack of membranes that envelops specific segments of neuronal axons within the nervous system [1]. Myelin in the central nervous system (CNS) is produced by oligodendrocytes (OLs). In contrast, the peripheral nervous system (PNS) relies on Schwann cells for this function [1, 2]. This membrane structure is among the most remarkable in the body; it is distinguished by a unique composition of lipids and proteins, setting it apart from typical cellular membranes [2–4]. In contrast to conventional cell membranes, it comprises of a higher proportion of lipids (≈75%) and a lower proportion of proteins (≈25%) [1–3]. Galactosylceramides and sulfatides, comprising of long-chain fatty acid groups, are the most typical myelin lipids. The high proportion of saturated, long-chain fatty acids exerts a significant impact on membrane structure, thereby influencing parameters such as myelin thickness and the packing density of lipids within myelin [2].

The discovery and understanding of myelin evolved over several centuries [5]. The first documented instance of the term "white matter" is attributed to Vesalius in the sixteenth century, while the observation of myelinated fibers is believed to have been made by van Leeuwenhoek in 1717. Notable contributions to this field include Remak's axon theory (1836), Schwann's description of nuclei (1839), and Virchow's coinage of the term "myelin" in 1854. In 1872, Ranvier proposed the hypothesis that myelin originated from fatty cells, which would subsequently be recognized as Schwann cells [5]. The term "oligodendrocytes" was coined by del Río-Hortega in 1919 and formally defined in 1921 [5]. Subsequent research, notably that of Penfield in 1924, established these cells as equivalent to Schwann cells within the CNS. The twentieth century saw significant progress in the understanding of myelin, with its fatty composition, crystal-like structure, and functional role in saltatory conduction being clarified in 1954 [5]. Subsequent electron microscopic analysis provided the initial evidence supporting the hypothesis that Schwann cells envelop axons, thereby forming compact myelin spirals. The central origin of myelin was subsequently elucidated, as OLs are distinctly located away from axons; in 1962, Bunge provided definitive evidence that OLs are responsible for myelin production [5].

In view of the advances made in the field of cellular and molecular biology, subsequent research has focused on the molecular mechanisms of OL development and myelination, which have consequently become central topics in glial research [2]. A wide range of models, including human, rodent, zebrafish, Xenopus, and non-human primates, has been employed to study myelination. For a considerable period, OLs and other glial cells were regarded as a basic "support system." However, recent advancements have prompted a reevaluation of these cells, leading to their recognition as active and essential participants within the CNS. The complex interactions among OLs, other glial cells, and neurons are now recognized as being critical for optimal brain function [2, 4, 6].

In the CNS, myelin and OLs are affected in several conditions (**Figure 1**) [7]. Myelin is a particularly susceptible target of CNS injuries, including hypoxia and ischemic stroke [2, 7]. However, the most prevalent pathology associated with OLs and myelin is MS, an inflammatory disease that predominantly affects young individuals worldwide [2]. It manifests with a higher frequency in women than in men, and the etiology of the disease is only partially understood. The current hypothesis is that genetic and environmental factors contribute to the development of MS [1, 2]. The immune system attacks OLs and myelin, and the CNS often fails to repair this damage, ultimately resulting in neuronal degeneration and severe disabilities [2]. Another group of disorders associated with myelin is referred to as leukodystrophies. While they have generally been regarded as genetic anomalies resulting in hypomyelination or demyelination, only a limited number of the implicated genes are exclusively expressed in OLs [1, 2].

Recent evidence highlights the active involvement of OLs and myelin in Alzheimer's disease (AD). Despite the established knowledge that myelin is subject to alterations during the process of aging, the prevailing paradigm regarding OLs has historically portrayed them as passive entities within the context of AD pathogenesis [8]. However, new findings indicate that there is a functional shift in the orientation of OLs towards a disease-associated state in response to amyloid and tau lesions [8]. Rather than being inert, they play a dual role in AD pathogenesis, on the one hand providing potential protective responses against pathology, while on the other hand contributing to disease progression [8].

Myelin has also been implicated in neurodevelopmental and psychiatric disorders, including autism spectrum disorder (ASD) and schizophrenia [9]. It is noteworthy that rodent models displaying ASD mutations exclusively in oligodendroglia exhibit certain phenotypes that mirror those observed in individuals with ASD [10].

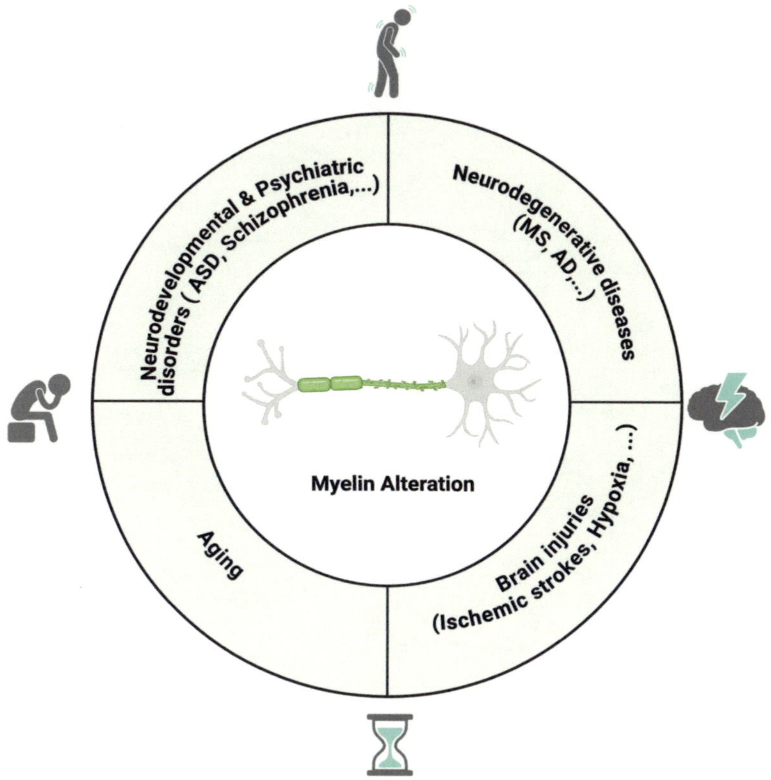

Figure 1.
Circular schematic illustrating that myelin alteration is a shared process across multiple CNS disorders. At the center is a drawing of a myelinated axon. Surrounding it is a ring divided into four segments representing: neurodegenerative diseases (e.g., multiple sclerosis (MS), Alzheimer's disease (AD), brain injuries (e.g., ischemic stroke, hypoxia), aging, and neurodevelopmental and psychiatric disorders (e.g., ASD, schizophrenia). Small icons around the circle symbolize the clinical or biological features associated with each category(adapted from [7]).

Here, we present a comprehensive overview of the mechanisms underlying myelination in the CNS and the key roles played by oligodendroglial cells across different contexts. While the primary focus of this review is on the CNS, occasional references to the PNS are included when structural or functional aspects of myelin are considered. Additionally, the emerging concept of myelin plasticity in the CNS is discussed, as it has become a major focus of research in the field [4, 6].

2. The journey from OPCs to myelin

OLs are derived from oligodendrocyte precursor cells (OPCs), which themselves originate from neural stem cells (NSCs) [1]. During the developmental process, OPCs undergo a series of changes that result in their differentiation into pre-myelinating OLs (**Figure 2**). These cells subsequently reach full maturity and functionality as fully mature OLs [1, 2], which extend processes that contact axons and generate the myelin sheath (**Figure 2**).

In the rodent cortex, OPCs emerge from the neuroepithelial regions surrounding the ventricles and are generated in three distinct developmental waves

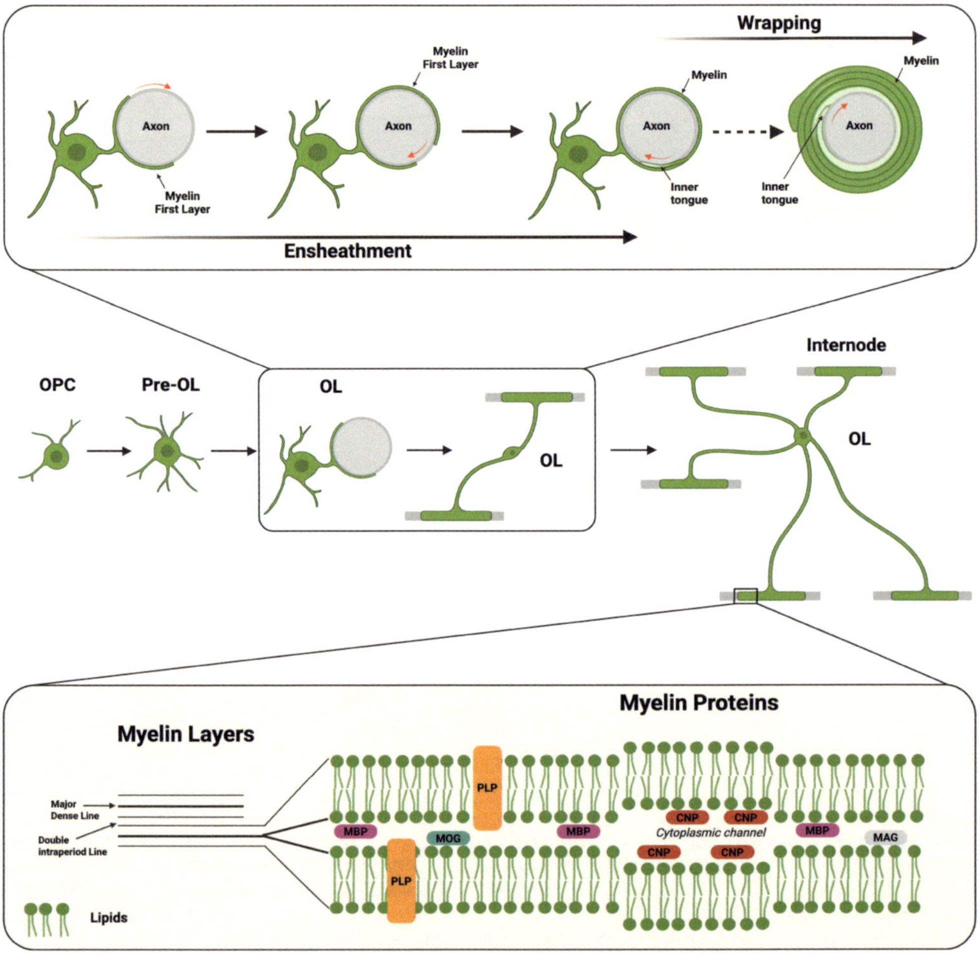

Figure 2.
Diagram illustrating oligodendroglia lineage and myelin structure. The top panel shows the steps of myelin formation, beginning with an oligodendrocyte extending its membrane around an axon, followed by progressive wrapping driven by the inner tongue to form a multilamellar myelin sheath. The middle panel depicts the differentiation of oligodendrocyte progenitor cells (OPCs) into pre-oligodendrocytes and then mature oligodendrocytes, which extend multiple processes to form internodes along several axons. The bottom panel shows a magnified view of compact myelin layers and their molecular components, including lipids and key proteins: MBP (magenta) promoting compaction, PLP (orange) and MOG (cyan) contributing to structural stability, MAG (gray) mediating axon–glia signaling, and CNP (red) maintaining cytoplasmic channels(adapted from [2]).

(E12.5, E15.5, and P0). It has been observed that these waves originate in the ventral region and progressively shift toward the dorsal regions [11, 12]. The OPCs from the first wave are predominantly replaced by medial and dorsal OPCs by postnatal day 10 (P10) [11]. In the spinal cord, two waves are identified: a ventral wave commencing at E12.5, which generates 80–90% of the total OPC population, and a dorsal wave that contributes the remaining 10–20% [13].

Once generated, OPCs migrate toward their target regions, guided by gradients of signaling molecules, extracellular matrix proteins (e.g., laminin, fibronectin), axon guidance cues (e.g., netrin-1, CXCL1), and growth factors such as vascular endothelial growth factor (VEGF) and platelet-derived growth factor (PDGF) [13].

Moreover, it has been shown that neuronal activity can promote OPC migration [14]. OPCs have been shown to express AMPA and NMDA receptors and to receive direct synaptic input from neurons [14, 15]. This finding lends support to the hypothesis that neurotransmitter release may function as a positional cue during migration. Furthermore, OPCs frequently migrate along blood vessels, using these vessels as structural "tracks" that facilitate the migration of OPCs between regions [16].

Upon reaching their destination, OPCs proliferate and differentiate [13]. The progression of these cells into pre-myelinating OLs and then into mature OLs is influenced by the activity of differentiation-promoting transcription factors, including myelin regulatory factor (Myrf). Mature OLs have been shown to initiate myelin production by expressing key myelin proteins, including MOG, MBP, and PLP. Together, these proteins facilitate the assembly of myelin sheaths, forming a compact bilayer lipid membrane that insulates and protects axons [13]. Myelin compaction is primarily mediated by MBP, which acts as a "zippering" protein between adjacent bilayer membranes [2, 17]. The process of MBP mRNA transport along microtubules from the OL soma to its processes, followed by on-site protein synthesis, is referred to as local translation [18]. It has been demonstrated that MBP exhibits a high degree of affinity for phosphatidylinositol-4,5-bisphosphate (PIP_2), a lipid constituent of the membrane [19]. The binding and neutralization of two PIP2 molecules by MBP result in the convergence of opposing bilayers, thereby forming the major dense line (**Figure 2**) and extruding cytoplasm from the space between them [20, 21]. PLP, a transmembrane protein, contributes to the adhesion of the extracellular leaflets of the myelin membrane (double intraperiod line, **Figure 2**), thereby further stabilizing the compact structure [21]. Mice deficient in PLP can still form compact myelin; however, the sheaths are physically unstable [22]. Despite its compaction, myelin facilitates the exchange of metabolites through cytoplasmic channels that are maintained by 2′,3′-cyclic nucleotide 3′ -phosphodiesterase (CNP). CNP counteracts MBP-mediated compaction by binding actin and creating intracellular "pillars" that maintain open, narrow cytoplasmic spaces [23]. These channels are more abundant in young animals than in adults [24] and enable the transport of metabolites, vesicles, and trophic molecules to the periaxonal space, supporting axo-glial unit maintenance [2]. Other myelin proteins, such as myelin oligodendrocyte glycoprotein (MOG) and myelin-associated glycoprotein (MAG), have also been shown to contribute to the stability and integrity of the sheath [25, 26].

Myelin formation exemplifies a particularly dramatic instance of morphological change in a living cell [27, 28]. OLs are subject to a process of extensive cytoskeletal remodeling, which is necessary for the extension of their processes, the wrapping of their axons, and the production of myelin. During OL development, the process of actin polymerization has been shown to drive outgrowth, branching, and ensheathment [27, 28]. Conversely, the process of wrapping during myelination requires the disassembly of actin. Despite the broad consensus on the necessity of actin depolymerization, the precise dynamics of this process remain a subject of debate. A body of research posits a continuous cycle of turnover of polymerization and depolymerization as the underlying mechanism that generates the forces necessary for the process of wrapping [27]. In contrast, other studies propose that depolymerization occurs only once at the onset of wrapping [28]. A recent study found that the transition from actin polymerization to depolymerization requires inhibition of the P21-Activated Kinase 1 (PAK1), mediated by the binding of the NF2/Merlin protein [29]. These findings reveal the fascinating antagonistic interplay between the pro-oncogenic kinase PAK1 and the tumor suppressor NF2/Merlin in myelin membrane expansion.

Microtubules (MTs), the other major component of the cytoskeleton in OLs, also play critical roles in myelination. These structures can be categorized into two distinct types: radial MTs, which extend toward processes, and lamellar MTs, which spiral longitudinally around the myelin sheath and traverse cytoplasmic channels [24]. The function of MTs is critical for the transport of mRNA and vesicles from the soma to the processes and within the myelin sheath (as noted above). Additionally, MTs are involved in process extension via polymerization and depolymerization dynamics [30]. Recent research has demonstrated that the nucleation of MTs outside the cell body is essential for the process of myelination. In particular, tubulin polymerization-promoting protein (TPPP) has been shown to mediate MT nucleation at Golgi outposts within OL processes [31]. The *in vivo* studies on TPPP depletion havent revealed that TPPP-deficient mice exhibit shorter and thinner myelin sheaths, along with motor coordination deficits on the rotarod test [31].

The CNS is a highly complex network comprising a diverse array of neuronal types with varying morphologies and sizes across different brain regions. Even within a single region, an OL may encounter multiple neuron types that vary in axonal diameter and function. Yet, the OL exhibits the capacity to selectively myelinate certain axons while leaving others unmyelinated [3]. OLs possess an intrinsic capacity to form myelin, with the ability to generate up to 80 sheaths on different axons [2]. In the PNS, axons with diameters greater than 1 μm are typically myelinated [32]. In contrast, the process of CNS myelination does not appear to adhere to such a rigid size criterion. For instance, in specific brain regions, axons measuring as small as 200–300 nm in diameter are myelinated, while in other regions, these axons remain unmyelinated [3]. Specific biophysical cues have been shown to influence the permissiveness of axons to myelination. In zebrafish, the first axon to be myelinated is the large-caliber Mauthner axon, and the generation of additional Mauthner axons alters how individual OLs allocate their myelinating capacity [33]. *In vitro*, axonal geometry has been demonstrated to influence OL behavior. Specifically, high-curvature surfaces have been demonstrated to be non-permissive, while large-diameter, low-curvature axons have been observed to promote myelination [34]. Increasing the diameter of normally unmyelinated cerebellar granule cell axons *in vitro* has been demonstrated to be sufficient to trigger myelination [35]. These findings suggest that, as in the PNS, large axons in the CNS may present cues that attract OLs. However, it is important to emphasize that axonal size, in isolation, does not serve as a definitive indicator of a specific condition. Molecular cues have been demonstrated to play a role in this process. In the PNS, neuregulin 1 (Nrg1) has been demonstrated to be sufficient to attract Schwann cells and initiate myelination; however, in the CNS, Nrg1 disruption does not block myelination, suggesting that multiple cues are involved [13, 34].

Furthermore, emerging evidence has demonstrated the critical function of neuronal activity in directing OL targeting. Indeed, studies of the zebrafish spinal cord have revealed that the inhibition of action potentials (AP) or activity-dependent vesicle release results in a reduction of myelination in specific axons [36, 37]. The release of glutamate has been identified as a mediator of this effect *in vitro* [38], although the precise receptor subtypes involved remain to be elucidated. The occurrence of activity-dependent regulation is not uniform; some neurons control myelin targeting in one brain region but not in another [39]. It is noteworthy that neurons are not completely myelinated, as OLs generally avoid myelinating dendrites and the soma [40]. Furthermore, in the adult CNS, a significant number of axons persist in an unmyelinated state or exhibit discontinuous or incomplete myelination, even in the presence of OLs [41]. These observations suggest the potential involvement of repulsive signals. Eph–ephrin interactions have been demonstrated to induce OL process retraction and reduce myelination [42, 43]. Polysialylated neural cell adhesion molecule (PSA-NCAM) has also been demonstrated to exert repulsive effects, with increased myelination resulting from its blocking and decreased myelination resulting from its overexpression [44, 45]. Recent findings indicate that junctional adhesion molecule 2 (Jam2) functions as an inhibitory cue, restricting myelination of the somatodendritic compartment [46]. In summary, OL axonal selection is likely governed by an integrated code of biophysical properties, attractive molecular signals, repulsive cues, and both activity-dependent and activity-independent mechanisms. The relative contribution of each factor is likely to vary according to brain region, neuron type, and even local microenvironment, and the same cue may exert different effects in different contexts [13].

3. Functions of oligodendroglial cells and myelin

The primary function of myelin is to increase the speed of AP propagation along axons. Myelinated segments (internodes, **Figure 2**) are interrupted by short unmyelinated regions known as the nodes of Ranvier, which are flanked by paranodes and juxtaparanodes [2] (**Figure 3**). The nodes, defined as the gaps between two internodes, have been observed to contain a high density of voltage-gated sodium channels, predominantly the Nav1.6 isoform, within the adult mammalian nervous system [47]. Furthermore, they have been found to harbor other ion channels, including Kv7.2/Kv7.3 voltage-gated potassium channels, which have been demonstrated to contribute to the stabilization of the resting membrane potential, as well as Kv3.1b channels, which have been shown to facilitate high-frequency firing [47]. In juxtaparanodes, there is a high density of delayed rectifier voltage-gated potassium channels (Kv1.1, Kv1.2) along with their auxiliary subunit Kvβ2. It is hypothesized that these channels and subunits contribute to maintaining the internodal resting potential [47]. The paranodes, which are devoid of ion channel clusters, are nevertheless essential for axon–glia junctions. At this site, a tight adhesion is formed between the myelin sheath and the axolemma. Neurofascin-155 (Nfasc155) on the myelin membrane interacts with Caspr 1 and contactin on the axolemma [48]. Consequently, nodes of Ranvier have been shown to facilitate rapid propagation of APs and stabilize axon-glia units by segregating ion channels into non-myelinated spots and establishing thight interaction with axolemma. In saltatory conduction, the AP effectively "jumps" from one node of Ranvier to the next, while the high compaction of the myelin sheath prevents ionic leak that could disrupt signal propagation, thereby optimizing CNS conductivity (**Figure 3**).

The other essential function of OLs and myelin is their role in providing metabolic support to neurons (**Figure 3**). Experimental studies have identified a lactate transporter in the innermost layer of myelin, positioned in close proximity to the axon [2, 49, 50]. Blocking this pathway leads to hypomyelination and axonal degeneration, underscoring the essential role of lactate transfer from OLs in sustaining myelinated neurons. This metabolic coupling necessitates the sensing of axonal activity by OLs [49]. Accordingly, glutamate receptors have been identified in the innermost layer of brain myelin [49]. Activation of these receptors has been shown to promote GLUT1 trafficking to the outer myelin and paranodal regions, thereby increasing glucose uptake and enhancing lactate delivery to active axons [49].

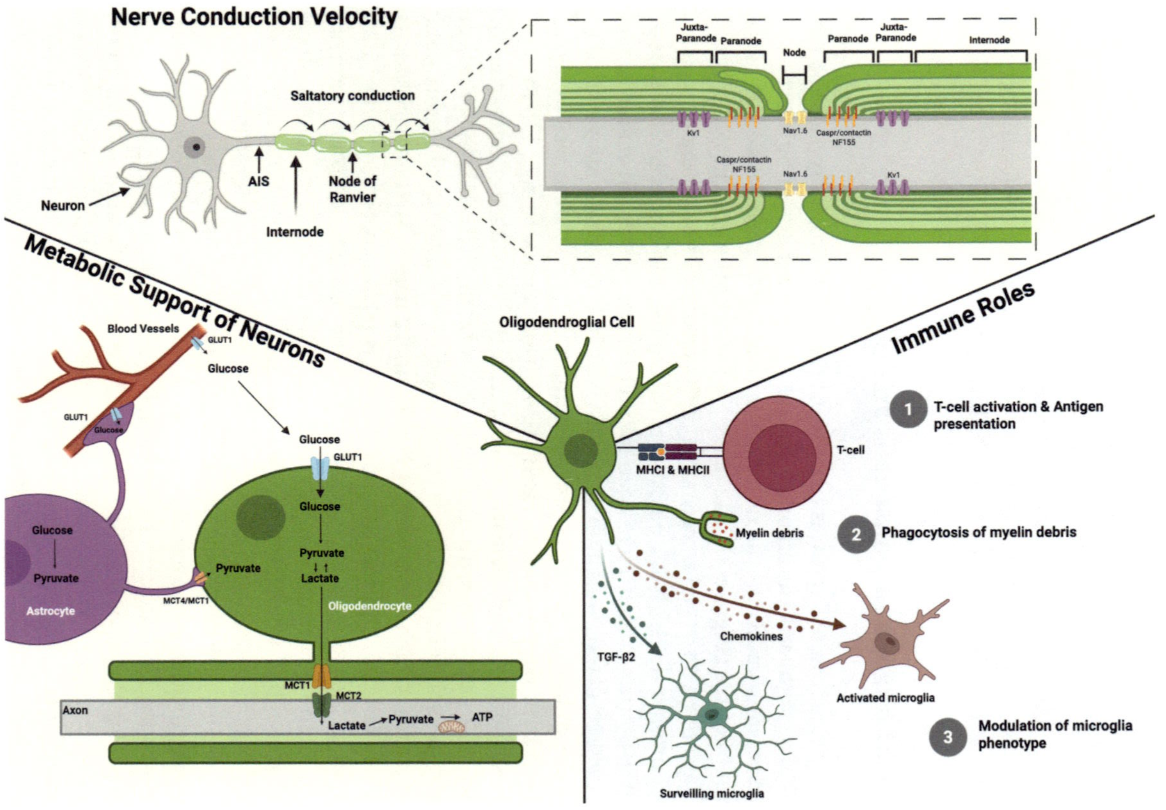

Figure 3.
Composite diagram illustrating three major functions of oligodendroglial cells and myelin. The top section shows nerve conduction velocity, with a myelinated axon displaying saltatory conduction between nodes of Ranvier. A magnified view highlights molecular specialization of axonal domains: Nav1.6 sodium channels at the node, NF155–Caspr/contactin complexes at paranodes, and Kv1 potassium channels at juxtaparanodes. The lower left section depicts metabolic support, showing glucose uptake from blood vessels and astrocytes via GLUT1, its conversion to pyruvate and lactate in oligodendrocytes, and transfer of lactate to axons through MCT1 (oligodendrocytes) and MCT2 (axons) to fuel ATP production. The right section illustrates immune roles of oligodendroglial cells: antigen presentation and T-cell activation via MHC molecules, phagocytosis of myelin debris, and modulation of microglial phenotype through chemokine release. (adapted from [51]).

While oligodendroglial cells (OPCs and OLs) are predominantly recognized for their role in myelination, numerous studies over the past years have highlighted their involvement in immune functions [51] (**Figure 3**). Within the CNS, the immune response is primarily orchestrated by microglia, the resident immune cells of the brain [2]. These cells perpetually survey their environment, poised to respond to injury or the intrusion of foreign substances.

OPCs have the capacity for phagocytosis, which serves to clear away debris, and they can also release cytokines, orchestrating responses in other cells [52]. OPCs exhibit several features that are analogous to those of microglia, including motility, phagocytic activity, and the capacity to respond to and release cytokines [52]. In vitro, primary rat OPCs have been demonstrated to phagocytose a variety of cellular debris, including myelin fragments and even cell membranes derived from astrocyte cultures [53]. *In vivo* evidence has emerged demonstrating the presence of axonal fragments and phagosomes within OPCs. Single-nucleus RNA sequencing data have revealed the expression of key phagocytic genes in OPCs, suggesting a potential role in brain shaping during development [54]. Beyond the clearance of debris, OPCs have also been demonstrated to contribute to the maintenance of CNS homeostasis under physiological conditions [51]. This process is facilitated by the release of TGF-β2, which has been shown to upregulate the microglial receptor CX3CR1 and promote a neuroprotective phenotype in microglia [55]. It has been demonstrated that depletion of NG2 glial cells consistently reduces the microglial homeostatic signature, leading to heightened activation and increased production of pro-inflammatory factors such as interleukin (IL)-1β, IL-6, and tumor necrosis factor (TNF) [56].

While oligodendroglial cells have not heretofore been regarded as a component of the immune system, OPCs have been demonstrated to exhibit a response to inflammation. In both human MS tissue [57] and mouse models [58], OPCs have been observed to express genes involved in antigen processing and presentation. These cells have been shown to produce a variety of inflammatory molecules, including cytokines and major histocompatibility complex (MHC) proteins. These molecules have been found to be upregulated in inflammatory contexts such as MS or experimental autoimmune encephalomyelitis (EAE) [59, 60]. *In vivo,* oligodendroglia expressing MHC class I and class II molecules have been shown to engage CD4 + and CD8 + T cells that have been previously activated [61]. In MS lesions, OPC numbers are reduced, potentially due to these interactions, which may enhance CD8 + T cell-mediated killing of OLs as well as CD4 + T cell-mediated cytotoxicity [61].

Similarly, the ablation of the oligodendroglial TNF receptor 2 (TNFR2) in EAE models exacerbates the immunomodulatory and inflammatory functions of OPCs following stimulation [62]. Collectively, these findings emphasize the multifaceted immunological functions of oligodendroglial cells and underscore their importance in understanding inflammatory myelin-related diseases, such as MS [51].

4. Myelin plasticity

Cerebral plasticity, also referred to as adaptive neural capacity, is defined as the brain's ability to modify its functions in response to processes such as learning. This capacity enables the brain to stabilize these modifications through homeostatic mechanisms and to restore functions following injury. While previous research indicated that this adaptability was exclusively attributable to neurons, recent studies have identified a growing body of evidence indicating the involvement of glial cells, particularly OLs and the myelin they produce [4, 6, 63]. MRI studies in humans have shown that learning can change the profile of white matter [64, 65]. Indeed, it has been demonstrated that the practice of piano, juggling, or the acquisition of reading skills and new languages are all associated with an increase in white matter volume (**Figure 4**). While this does not provide direct evidence of myelin remodeling, it strongly suggests its involvement. Rodent models have played a particularly instrumental role in elucidating the adaptive properties of myelin. The findings that the adult CNS is not fully myelinated, that individual neurons can display intermittent myelination with unmyelinated segments [41], and that OPCs remain abundant in the adult brain [66], collectively suggest that new myelin can still be generated. A concrete example that clearly suggests myelin could serve as a means of circuit adaptation is the myelination of the neuronal circuit controlling binaural hearing, which enables sound localization [67]. A differential pattern of myelination has been observed between the ipsilateral and contralateral branches of brainstem cochlear nucleus neurons. This differential profile ensures faster signal

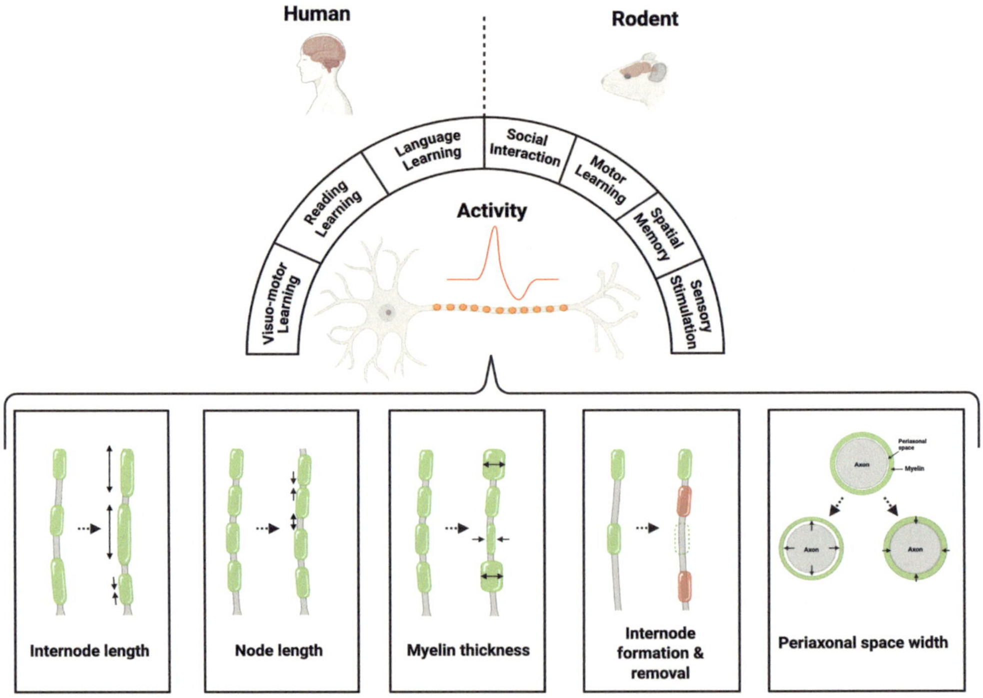

Figure 4.
Diagram illustrating activity-dependent white-matter and myelin plasticity in humans and rodents. The upper panel shows that neuronal activity, driven by behaviors such as visuomotor learning, reading, and language acquisition in humans, and by social interaction, motor learning, spatial memory, and sensory stimulation in rodents, induces adaptive myelin remodeling. The central illustration depicts an active neuron. The bottom panel highlights structural changes observed in myelinated axons, including modifications in internode length, node of Ranvier length, myelin thickness, internode formation or removal, and periaxonal space width.(adapted from [4]).

conduction along the more heavily myelinated contralateral branches, thereby compensating for their longer conduction path. Conduction velocity is contingent upon the degree of myelination, and adaptive myelination exerts a substantial influence on synaptic responses. For instance, it can synchronize the arrival times of electrical signals from different neurons onto a common postsynaptic target, thereby maximizing temporal summation. Consequently, adaptive myelination also addresses specific physiological requirements for the proper functioning of neuronal circuits.

Recent studies using genetic fate mapping have demonstrated that new OLs are indeed generated in the adult brain [66], and that their generation is activity-dependent, much like during development [68, 69]. Remarkably, *in vivo* two-photon imaging of the adult rodent cerebral cortex has demonstrated unequivocally that new myelin segments are generated during adulthood and that existing segments can both elongate and retract [4, 70, 71].

A seminal study revealed an increase in MBP density in the brain region responsible for motor task learning in rodents [72]. This suggests a correlation between MBP density and motor learning. Another team of researchers demonstrated that the inhibition of new OL generation impairs motor learning [73]. Therefore, the generation of newly formed OLs is necessary for motor learning. It has been shown that motor learning drives the early proliferation of OPCs in the motor cortex and the underlying white matter, with a fraction of them differentiating into myelinating OLs [74]. Recent investigations employing in vivo two-photon imaging have posited that myelin sheaths surrounding learning-activated axons initially retract during the learning process. This retraction leads to the formation of elongated nodes of Ranvier and a new pattern of sparse myelination on these axons [75]. This is believed to result in a transient reduction in conduction velocity during learning tasks [75]. In a subsequent phase, newly generated OLs form new myelin sheaths, preferentially positioned between the retracted existing sheaths [75]. This sequential process establishes a modified pattern of myelination along activated neurons, distinguished by addition of new myelin sheaths [75]. This remodeling has the potential to enhance conduction velocity, thereby facilitating the optimization of signal transmission along consolidated neural circuits following learning.

Memory training in mice also depends on the generation of new OLs [6]. In the water maze paradigm, spatial memory acquisition requires the production of new OLs specifically in the regions activated during training and the subsequent post-training period that supports consolidation [76]. Blocking OPC differentiation during training or consolidation impairs learning and increases latencies in remote recall tasks [76]. Similar results were obtained in contextual fear memory paradigms, in which successful memory formation required OPC proliferation, differentiation into OLs, and subsequent myelin generation [76, 77]. The temporal profile suggests that OPC proliferation and differentiation are crucial during the learning phase, while the formation of new myelin, which emerges weeks after training, plays a more prominent role in memory consolidation than in acute learning [77]. A recent in-depth analysis of oligodendroglial dynamics in spatial working memory tasks confirmed these observations [78]. Memory efficiency was closely linked to both early OPC proliferation and differentiation in stimulated regions and to the overall extent of these processes [78]. Memory consolidation involves subsequent structural remodeling, including the formation of shorter myelin internodes and the insertion of additional sheaths between existing ones [78]. These modifications are expected to increase conduction velocity and mirror the adaptive changes observed in motor learning [78].

Conversely, adverse environmental stimuli have been demonstrated to exert detrimental effects on myelination. In adult mice, social isolation has been demonstrated to induce impairments in social behavior and a reduction in social interest toward conspecifics [79]. In the prefrontal cortex (PFC), it has been reported that there is a global thinning of myelin sheaths, independent of axonal diameter. Reintegration of mice with congeners was able to restore myelin defects as well as social interactions [79]. Remarkably, pharmacological restoration of myelin with clemastine, a muscarinic agonist, was sufficient to rescue social deficits in isolated adult mice [80]. Importantly, social isolation of mice during the juvenile phase also leads to defects similar to those observed following isolation in adulthood [81]. Reintegration with other previously isolated mice does not rescue the defects [81], whereas reintegration with socially housed (non-isolated) animals does [82]. These findings emphasize the remarkable plasticity of myelin and its capacity to modulate cognitive behavior.

Strikingly, myelin plasticity manifests in various ways (**Figure 4**), including changes in internode length, thickness, and spacing, as well as alterations in the length of the nodes of Ranvier and the width of the periaxonal space, all of which influence neuronal physiology [4, 83].

5. Conclusion

Myelin is no longer regarded as a static structure; rather, it is recognized as a dynamic and adaptive structure capable of remodeling in response to electrical activity and experience. These properties underscore the critical role of myelin in both health and disease. Despite these advances, the molecular mechanisms underlying myelin plasticity remain largely unexplored, opening broad avenues of research that span molecular and cellular biology to membrane biophysics. Advancements in this field are expected to significantly improve our understanding of CNS function and the mechanisms that drive related disorders.

Acronyms and abbreviations

AMPA	Alpha-amino-3-hydroxy-5-methyl-4-isooxazole-propionic acid
AP	Action potential
Caspr 1	Contactin-associated protein 1
CNP	2′,3′-Cyclic nucleotide 3′-phosphodiesterase
CNS	Central nervous system
EAE	Experimental autoimmune encephalomyelitis
GLUT1	Glucose transporter 1
IL	Interleukin
Kv	Voltage-gated potassium
MAG	Myelin-associated glycoprotein
MBP	Myelin basic protein

DOI: http://dx.doi.org/10.5772/intechopen.1013216

MCT1	Monocarboxylate transporter 1
MCT2	Monocarboxylate transporter 2
MHC	Major histocompatibility complex
MOG	Myelin oligodendrocyte glycoprotein
MS	Multiple sclerosis
MT	Microtubule
MRI	Magnetic resonance imaging
Myrf	Myelin regulatory factor
Nav	Voltage-gated sodium
NFasc155	Neurofascin 155
NF2	Neurofibromatosis type II
NMDA	N-methyl-D-aspartate
Nrg1	Neuregulin 1
NSC	Neural stem cell
NT	Neurotransmitter
OL	Oligodendrocyte
OPC	Oligodendrocyte precursor Cell
PAK1	P21 activated kinase 1
PDGF	Platelet-derived growth factor
PFC	Prefrontal cortex
PIP2	Phosphatidylinositol-4,5-bisphosphate
PLP	Proteolipid protein
PNS	Peripheral nervous system
PSA-NCAM	Polysialylated neural cell adhesion molecule
RNA	Ribonucleic acid
TGF	Transforming growth factor
TNF	Tumor necrosis factor
TNFR2	Tumor necrosis factor receptor 2
TPPP	Tubulin polymerization promoting protein
VEGF	Vascular endothelial growth factor

Acknowledgments

We thank the Fondation France Sclérose en Plaques, the Fondation Jérôme Lejeune, and Sorbonne University for their financial support.

The figures were prepared using BioRender, and artificial intelligence was employed to refine and enhance the writing.

Conflict of interest

The authors declare no conflict of interest.

Author details

Julie Pilon[1,2] and Lamia Bouslama-Oueghlani[1,2*]

1 Sorbonne University, Paris, France

2 Paris cité University, Institute of Psychiatry and Neuroscience of Paris (IPNP), INSERM U1266, Paris, France

*Address all correspondence to: lamia.bouslama@sorbonne-universite.fr

References

[1] Baumann N, Pham-Dinh D. Biology of oligodendrocyte and myelin in the mammalian central nervous system. Physiological Reviews. 2001;**81**(2): 871–927

[2] Stadelmann C, Timmler S, Barrantes-Freer A, Simons M. Myelin in the central nervous system: Structure, function, and pathology. Physiological Reviews. 2019;**99**(3):1381–431. DOI: 10.1152/physrev.00031.2018

[3] Simons M, Lyons DA. Axonal selection and myelin sheath generation in the central nervous system. Current Opinion in Cell Biology. 2013;**25**(4): 512–9. DOI: 10.1016/j.ceb.2013.04.007

[4] Osso LA, Hughes EG. Dynamics of mature myelin. Nature Neuroscience. 2024;**27**(8):1449–61. DOI: 10.1038/s41593-024-01642-2

[5] Boullerne AI. The history of myelin. Experimental Neurology. 2016;**283** (Pt B):431–45. DOI: 10.1016/j.expneurol.2016.06.005

[6] Xin W, Chan JR. Myelin plasticity: Sculpting circuits in learning and memory. Nature Reviews Neuroscience. 2020. DOI: 10.1038/s41583-020-00379-8 **21** 682–694

[7] Huang Z, Zhang Y, Zou P, Zong X, Zhang Q. Myelin dysfunction in aging and brain disorders: Mechanisms and therapeutic opportunities. Molecular Neurodegeneration. 2025;**20**(1):69. DOI: 10.1186/s13024-025-00861-w

[8] Kedia S, Simons M. Oligodendrocytes in Alzheimer's disease pathophysiology. Nature Neuroscience. 2025;**28**(3):446–56. DOI: 10.1038/s41593-025-01873-x

[9] Khelfaoui H, Ibaceta-Gonzalez C, Angulo MC. Functional myelin in cognition and neurodevelopmental disorders. Cellular and Molecular Life Sciences: CMLS. 2024;**81**(1):181. DOI: 10.1007/s00018-024-05222-2

[10] Phan BDN, Bohlen JF, Davis BA, Ye Z, Chen HY, Mayfield B, et al. A myelin-related transcriptomic profile is shared by Pitt–Hopkins syndrome models and human autism spectrum disorder. Nature Neuroscience. 2020. DOI: 10.1038/s41593-019-0578-x. **23** 375–385

[11] Kessaris N, Fogarty M, Iannarelli P, Grist M, Wegner M, Richardson WD. Competing waves of oligodendrocytes in the forebrain and postnatal elimination of an embryonic lineage. Nature Neuroscience. 2006;**9**(2):173–9. DOI: 10.1038/nn1620

[12] Richardson WD, Kessaris N, Pringle N. Oligodendrocyte wars. Nature Reviews Neuroscience. 2006;**7** (1):11–8. DOI: 10.1038/nrn1826

[13] van Tilborg E, de Theije CGM, van Hal M, Wagenaar N, de Vries LS, Benders MJ, et al. Origin and dynamics of oligodendrocytes in the developing brain: Implications for perinatal white matter injury. Glia. 2018;**66**(2):221–228

[14] Moura DMS, Brennan EJ, Brock R, Cocas LA. Neuron to oligodendrocyte precursor cell synapses: Protagonists in Oligodendrocyte development and myelination, and targets for therapeutics. Frontiers in Neuroscience. 2022;**15**. DOI: 10.3389/fnins.2021.779125

[15] Karadottir R, Cavelier P, Bergersen LH, Attwell D. NMDA receptors are expressed in oligodendrocytes and activated in ischaemia. Nature. 2005;**438** (7071):1162–6. DOI: 10.1038/nature04302

[16] Tsai HH, Niu J, Munji R, Davalos D, Chang J, Zhang H, et al. Oligodendrocyte precursors migrate along vasculature in the developing nervous system. Science. 2016;**351** (6271):379–84. DOI: 10.1126/science.aad3839

[17] Nave K-A, Werner HB. Myelination of the Nervous System: Mechanisms and functions. Annual Review of Cell and Developmental Biology. 2014. DOI: 10.1146/annurev-cellbio-100913-013101. **30** 503–533

[18] Barbarese E, Brumwell C, Kwon S, Cui H, Carson JH. RNA on the road to myelin. Journal of Neurocytology. 1999;**28**(4-5):263–70. DOI: 10.1023/a:1007097226688

[19] Nawaz S, Kippert A, Saab AS, Werner HB, Lang T, Nave KA, et al. Phosphatidylinositol 4,5-bisphosphate-dependent interaction of myelin basic protein with the plasma membrane in oligodendroglial cells and its rapid perturbation by elevated calcium. The Journal of Neuroscience. 2009;**29** (15):4794–807. DOI: 10.1523/JNEUROSCI.3955-08.2009

[20] Aggarwal S, Snaidero N, Pähler G, Frey S, Sánchez P, Zweckstetter M, et al. Myelin membrane assembly is driven by a phase transition of myelin basic proteins into a cohesive protein meshwork. PLoS Biology. 2013;**11**(6): e1001577. DOI: 10.1371/journal.pbio.1001577

[21] Aggarwal S, Yurlova L, Snaidero N, Reetz C, Frey S, Zimmermann J, et al. A size barrier limits protein diffusion at the cell surface to generate lipid-rich myelin-membrane sheets. Developmental Cell. 2011;**21**(3):445–56. DOI: 10.1016/j.devcel.2011.08.001

[22] Klugmann M, Schwab MH, Pühlhofer A, Schneider A, Zimmermann F, Griffiths IR, et al. Assembly of CNS myelin in the absence of proteolipid protein. Neuron. 1997;**18** (1):59–70. DOI: 10.1016/s0896-6273(01)80046-5

[23] Snaidero N, Velte C, Myllykoski M, Raasakka A, Ignatev A, Werner HB, et al. Antagonistic functions of MBP and CNP establish cytosolic Channels in CNS Myelin. Cell Reports. 2017;**18** (2):314–23. DOI: 10.1016/j.celrep.2016.12.053

[24] Weigel M, Wang L, Fu M-m. Microtubule organization and dynamics in oligodendrocytes, astrocytes, and microglia. Developmental Neurobiology. 2021;**81**(3):310–20. DOI: 10.1002/dneu.22753

[25] Ambrosius W, Michalak S, Kozubski W, Kalinowska A. Myelin Oligodendrocyte Glycoprotein antibody-associated disease: Current insights into the disease pathophysiology, diagnosis and management. International Journal of Molecular Sciences. 2020;**22**(1). 20201224. DOI: 10.3390/ijms22010100

[26] Li C, Tropak MB, Gerlai R, Clapoff S, Abramow-Newerly W, Trapp B, et al. Myelination in the absence of myelin-associated glycoprotein. Nature. 1994;**369** (6483):747–50. DOI: 10.1038/369747a0

[27] Nawaz S, Sanchez P, Schmitt S, Snaidero N, Mitkovski M, Velte C, et al. Actin filament turnover drives leading edge growth during myelin sheath formation in the central nervous system. Developmental Cell. 2015;**34**(2):139–51. DOI: 10.1016/j.devcel.2015.05.013

[28] Zuchero JB, Fu MM, Sloan SA, Ibrahim A, Olson A, Zaremba A, et al. CNS myelin wrapping is driven by actin disassembly. Developmental Cell. 2015;**34**(2):152–67. DOI: 10.1016/j.devcel.2015.06.011

[29] Baudouin L, Ades N, Kante K, Bachelin C, Hmidan H, Deboux C, et al. Antagonistic actions of PAK1 and NF2/Merlin drive myelin membrane expansion in oligodendrocytes. Glia. 2024. e20240525. DOI: 10.1002/glia.24570

[30] Richter-Landsberg C. The cytoskeleton in oligodendrocytes. Microtubule dynamics in health and disease. Journal of Molecular Neuroscience. 2008;**35**(1):55–63. DOI: 10.1007/s12031-007-9017-7

[31] Fu M-M, McAlear TS, Nguyen H, Oses-Prieto JA, Valenzuela A, Shi RD, et al. The Golgi outpost protein TPPP nucleates microtubules and is critical for myelination. Cell. 2019;**179**(1):132–46.e14. DOI: 10.1016/j.cell.2019.08.025

[32] Sherman DL, Brophy PJ. Mechanisms of axon ensheathment and myelin growth. Nature Reviews Neuroscience. 2005;**6**(9):683–90. DOI: 10.1038/nrn1743

[33] Almeida RG, Czopka T, Ffrench-Constant C, Lyons DA. Individual axons regulate the myelinating potential of single oligodendrocytes in vivo. Development. 2011;**138**(20):4443–50. DOI: 10.1242/dev.071001

[34] Almeida RG. The rules of attraction in central nervous system myelination. Frontiers in Cellular Neuroscience. 2018;**12**:367. DOI: 10.3389/fncel.2018.00367

[35] Goebbels S, Wieser GL, Pieper A, Spitzer S, Weege B, Yan K, et al. A neuronal PI(3,4,5)P3-dependent program of oligodendrocyte precursor recruitment and myelination. Nature Neuroscience. 2017;**20**(1):10–5. DOI: 10.1038/nn.4425

[36] Hines JH, Ravanelli AM, Schwindt R, Scott EK, Appel B. Neuronal activity biases axon selection for myelination in vivo. Nature Neuroscience. 2015;**18**(5):683–9. DOI: 10.1038/nn.3992

[37] Mensch S, Baraban M, Almeida R, Czopka T, Ausborn J, El Manira A, et al. Synaptic vesicle release regulates myelin sheath number of individual oligodendrocytes in vivo. Nature Neuroscience. 2015;**18**(5):628–30. DOI: 10.1038/nn.3991

[38] Spitzer S, Volbracht K, Lundgaard I, Karadottir RT. Glutamate signalling: A multifaceted modulator of oligodendrocyte lineage cells in health and disease. Neuropharmacology. 2016;**110**(Pt B):574–85. DOI: 10.1016/j.neuropharm.2016.06.014

[39] Koudelka S, Voas MG, Almeida RG, Baraban M, Soetaert J, Meyer MP, et al. Individual neuronal subtypes exhibit diversity in CNS Myelination mediated by synaptic vesicle release. Current Biology. 2016;**26**(11):1447–55. DOI: 10.1016/j.cub.2016.03.070

[40] Lubetzki C, Demerens C, Anglade P, Villarroya H, Frankfurter A, Lee VM, Zalc B. Even in culture, oligodendrocytes myelinate solely axons. Proceedings of the National Academy of Sciences USA. 1993;**90**(14). DOI: 10.1016/j.neuron.2016.07.021

[41] Tomassy GS, Berger DR, Chen HH, Kasthuri N, Hayworth KJ, Vercelli A, et al. Distinct profiles of myelin distribution along single axons of pyramidal neurons in the neocortex. Science. 2014;**344**(6181):319–24. DOI: 10.1126/science.1249766

[42] Harboe M, Torvund-Jensen J, Kjaer-Sorensen K, Laursen LS. Ephrin-A1-EphA4 signaling negatively regulates myelination in the central nervous system. GLIA. 2018;**66**(5):934. DOI: 10.1002/glia.23293

[43] Linneberg C, Harboe M, Laursen LS. Axo-Glia interaction preceding CNS Myelination is regulated by Bidirectional Eph-Ephrin signaling. ASN Neuro. 2015;7(5). DOI: 10.1177/1759091415602859

[44] Charles P, Hernandez MP, Stankoff B, Aigrot MS, Colin C, Rougon G, et al. Negative regulation of central nervous system myelination by polysialylated-neural cell adhesion molecule. Proceedings of the National Academy of Sciences of the United States of America. 2000;**97**(13):7585–90. DOI: 10.1073/pnas.100076197

[45] Fewou SN, Ramakrishnan H, Bussow H, Gieselmann V, Eckhardt M. Down-regulation of polysialic acid is required for efficient myelin formation. Journal of Biological Chemistry. 2007;**282**(22):16700–11. DOI: 10.1074/jbc.M610797200

[46] Redmond SA, Mei F, Eshed-Eisenbach Y, Osso LA, Leshkowitz D, Shen Y-AA, et al. Somatodendritic expression of JAM2 inhibits Oligodendrocyte myelination. Neuron. 2016;**91**(4):824–36. DOI: 10.1016/j.neuron.2016.07.021

[47] Lubetzki C, Sol-Foulon N, Desmazieres A. Nodes of Ranvier during development and repair in the CNS. Nature Reviews Neurology. 2020;**16**(8):426–39. DOI: 10.1038/s41582-020-0375-x

[48] Ghosh A, Sherman DL, Brophy PJ. The Axonal Cytoskeleton and the assembly of nodes of Ranvier. The Neuroscientist. 2018;**24**(2):104–10. DOI: 10.1177/1073858417710897

[49] Saab AS, Tzvetavona ID, Trevisiol A, Baltan S, Dibaj P, Kusch K, et al. Oligodendroglial NMDA receptors regulate glucose import and axonal energy metabolism. Neuron. 2016;**91**(1):119–32. DOI: 10.1016/j.neuron.2016.05.016

[50] Lee Y, Morrison BM, Li Y, Lengacher S, Farah MH, Hoffman PN, et al. Oligodendroglia metabolically support axons and contribute to neurodegeneration. Nature. 2012;**487**(7408):443–8. DOI: 10.1038/nature11314

[51] Boccazzi M, Raffaele S, Fumagalli M. Not only myelination: The immune-inflammatory functions of oligodendrocytes. Neural Regeneration Research. 2022;**17**(12):2661–3. DOI: 10.4103/1673-5374.342678

[52] Haroon A, Seerapu H, Fang LP, Wess JH, Bai X. Unlocking the Potential: Immune functions of oligodendrocyte precursor cells.

Frontiers in Immunology. 2024;**15**:1425706. DOI: 10.3389/fimmu.2024.1425706

[53] Hamanaka G, Hernandez IC, Takase H, Ishikawa H, Benboujja F, Kimura S, et al. Myelination- and migration-associated genes are downregulated after phagocytosis in cultured oligodendrocyte precursor cells. Journal of Neurochemistry. 2023;**167**(4):571–81. DOI: 10.1111/jnc.15994

[54] Buchanan J, Elabbady L, Collman F, Jorstad NL, Bakken TE, Ott C, et al. Oligodendrocyte precursor cells ingest axons in the mouse neocortex. Proceedings of the National Academy of Sciences of the United States of America. 2022;**119**(48):e2202580119-e. DOI: 10.1073/pnas.2202580119

[55] Zhang SZ, Wang QQ, Yang QQ, Gu HY, Yin YQ, Li YD, et al. NG2 glia regulate brain innate immunity via TGF-beta2/TGFBR2 axis. BMC Medicine. 2019;**17**(1):204. DOI: 10.1016/j.expneurol.2016.06.005

[56] Nakano M, Tamura Y, Yamato M, Kume S, Eguchi A, Takata K, et al. NG2 glial cells regulate neuroimmunological responses to maintain neuronal function and survival. Scientific Reports. 2017;7:42041. DOI: 10.1038/srep42041

[57] Jakel S, Agirre E, Mendanha Falcao A, van Bruggen D, Lee KW, Knuesel I, et al. Altered human oligodendrocyte heterogeneity in multiple sclerosis. Nature. 2019;**566**(7745):543–7. DOI: 10.1038/s41586-019-0903-2

[58] Kirby L, Jin J, Cardona JG, Smith MD, Martin KA, Wang J, et al. Oligodendrocyte precursor cells present antigen and are cytotoxic targets in inflammatory demyelination. Nat Commun. 2019;**10**(1):3887. DOI: 10.1038/s41467-019-11638-3

[59] Falcão AM, van Bruggen D, Marques S, Meijer M, Jäkel S, Agirre E, et al. Disease-specific oligodendrocyte lineage cells arise in multiple sclerosis. Nature Medicine. 2018;**24**(12):1837–44. DOI: 10.1038/s41591-018-0236-y

[60] Schirmer L, Velmeshev D, Holmqvist S, Kaufmann M, Werneburg S, Jung D, et al. Neuronal vulnerability and multilineage diversity in multiple sclerosis. Nature. 2019;**573**(7772):75–82. DOI: 10.1038/s41586-019-1404-z

[61] Harrington EP, Bergles DE, Calabresi PA. Immune cell modulation of oligodendrocyte lineage cells. Neuroscience Letters. 2020;**715**:134601. DOI: 10.1016/j.neulet.2019.134601

[62] Desu HL, Illiano P, Choi JS, Ascona MC, Gao H, Lee JK, et al. TNFR2 signaling regulates the immunomodulatory function of Oligodendrocyte precursor cells. Cells. 2021;**10**(7). DOI: 10.3390/cells10071785.1785

[63] Baudouin L, Ades N, Bouslama-Oueghlani L. [Myelin: A new player in brain plasticity]. Médecine/sciences. 2021;**37**(5):535–8. DOI: 10.1051/medsci/2021045

[64] de Faria O, Jr., Pivonkova H, Varga B, Timmler S, Evans KA, Karadottir RT. Periods of synchronized myelin changes shape brain function and plasticity. Nature Neuroscience. 2021;**24**(11):1508–21. DOI: 10.1038/s41593-021-00917-2

[65] Fields RD. A new mechanism of nervous system plasticity: Activity-dependent myelination. Nature Reviews Neuroscience. 2015;**16**(12):756–67. DOI: 10.1038/nrn4023

[66] Young KM, Psachoulia K, Tripathi RB, Dunn SJ, Cossell L, Attwell D, et al. Oligodendrocyte dynamics in the healthy adult CNS: Evidence for myelin remodeling. Neuron. 2013;**77**(5):873–85. DOI: 10.1016/j.neuron.2013.01.006

[67] Seidl AH. Regulation of conduction time along axons. Neuroscience. 2014;**276**:126–34. DOI: 10.1016/j.neuroscience.2013.06.047

[68] Gibson EM, Purger D, Mount CW, Goldstein AK, Lin GL, Wood LS, et al. Neuronal activity promotes oligodendrogenesis and adaptive myelination in the mammalian brain. Science. 2014;**344**(6183):1252304. DOI: 10.1126/science.1252304

[69] Mitew S, Gobius I, Fenlon LR, McDougall SJ, Hawkes D, Xing YL, et al. Pharmacogenetic stimulation of neuronal activity increases myelination in an axon-specific manner. Nature Communications. 2018;**9**(1):306. DOI: 10.1038/s41467-017-02719-2

[70] Hughes EG, Orthmann-Murphy JL, Langseth AJ, Bergles DE. Myelin remodeling through experience-dependent oligodendrogenesis in the adult somatosensory cortex. Nature Neuroscience. 2018;**21**(5):696–706. DOI: 10.1038/s41593-018-0121-5

[71] Hill RA, Li AM, Grutzendler J. Lifelong cortical myelin plasticity and age-related degeneration in the live mammalian brain. Nature Neuroscience. 2018;**21**(5):683–95. DOI: 10.1038/s41593-018-0120-6

[72] Sampaio-Baptista C, Khrapitchev AA, Foxley S, Schlagheck T, Scholz J, Jbabdi S, et al. Motor skill learning induces changes in white matter microstructure and myelination. The Journal of Neuroscience. 2013;**33**(50):19499–503. DOI: 10.1523/JNEUROSCI.3048-13.2013

[73] McKenzie IA, Ohayon D, Li H, de Faria JP, Emery B, Tohyama K, et al. Motor skill learning requires active central myelination. Science. 2014;**346**(6207):318–22. DOI: 10.1126/science.1254960

[74] Xiao L, Ohayon D, McKenzie IA, Sinclair-Wilson A, Wright JL, Fudge AD, et al. Rapid production of new oligodendrocytes is required in the earliest stages of motor-skill learning. Nature Neuroscience. 2016;**19**(9):1210–7. DOI: 10.1038/nn.4351

[75] Bacmeister CM, Huang R, Osso LA, Thornton MA, Conant L, Chavez AR, et al. Motor learning drives dynamic patterns of intermittent myelination on learning-activated axons. Nature Neuroscience. 2022;**25**(10):1300–13. DOI: 10.1038/s41593-022-01169-4

[76] Steadman PE, Xia F, Ahmed M, Mocle AJ, Penning ARA, Geraghty AC, et al. Disruption of Oligodendrogenesis Impairs Memory Consolidation in Adult Mice. Neuron. 2020;**105**(1):150–64 e6. DOI: 10.1016/j.neuron.2019.10.013

[77] Pan S, Mayoral SR, Choi HS, Chan JR, Kheirbek MA. Preservation of a remote fear memory requires new myelin formation. Nature

Neuroscience. 2020;**23**(4):487–99. DOI: 10.1038/s41593-019-0582-1

[78] Shimizu T, Nayar SG, Swire M, Jiang Y, Grist M, Kaller M, et al. Oligodendrocyte dynamics dictate cognitive performance outcomes of working memory training in mice. Nature Communications. 2023;**14**(1):6499. DOI: 10.1038/s41467-023-42293-4

[79] Liu J, Dietz K, DeLoyht JM, Pedre X, Kelkar D, Kaur J, et al. Impaired adult myelination in the prefrontal cortex of socially isolated mice. Nature Neuroscience. 2012;**15**(12):1621–3. DOI: 10.1038/nn.3263

[80] Liu J, Dupree JL, Gacias M, Frawley R, Sikder T, Naik P, et al. Clemastine enhances Myelination in the prefrontal cortex and rescues behavioral changes in socially isolated mice. The Journal of Neuroscience. 2016;**36**(3):957–62. DOI: 10.1523/JNEUROSCI.3608-15.2016

[81] Makinodan M, Rosen KM, Ito S, Corfas G. A critical period for social experience-dependent oligodendrocyte maturation and myelination. Science. 2012;**337**(6100):1357–60. DOI: 10.1126/science.1220845

[82] Makinodan M, Ikawa D, Yamamuro K, Yamashita Y, Toritsuka M, Kimoto S, et al. Effects of the mode of re-socialization after juvenile social isolation on medial prefrontal cortex myelination and function. Scientific Reports. 2017. DOI: 10.1038/s41598-017-05632-2. 7

[83] Cullen CL, Pepper RE, Clutterbuck MT, Pitman KA, Oorschot V, Auderset L, et al. Periaxonal and nodal plasticities modulate action potential conduction in the adult mouse brain. Cell Reports. 2021;**34**(3):108641. DOI: 10.1016/j.celrep.2020.108641

Section 4

Reactive Astrocytes and Repair

Chapter 4

Proliferative Reactive Astrocytes: Key Regulators of Repair and Synaptic Remodeling in the Injured CNS

Lilesh Kumar Pradhan and Xiang Gao

Abstract

Following injury to the central nervous system (CNS), astrocytes, normally supportive glial cells, undergo a transformation into a reactive state. Among these, a distinct subset known as proliferative reactive astrocytes emerges and plays a critical role in both injury response and tissue repair. This topic explores the complex functions of these astrocytes beyond glial scar formation, highlighting their involvement in neuroprotection, synaptic remodeling, and the restoration of CNS homeostasis. Proliferative reactive astrocytes are regulated by signaling pathways such as JAK/STAT3, Notch, and YAP/TAZ, which control their activation, proliferation, and interaction with other cell types. These astrocytes engage closely with neurons, microglia, and the extracellular matrix, influencing inflammatory responses, axon regeneration, and synaptic plasticity. Their behavior is not uniform; rather, it shows significant regional and temporal heterogeneity, suggesting that their function is finely tuned to the injury context. Understanding the roles of proliferative astrocytes is essential for developing targeted therapies for CNS injuries and neurodegenerative diseases. Instead of being solely seen as barriers to regeneration, these cells are now recognized as potential agents of repair. Emerging strategies aim to modulate their behavior to enhance recovery while minimizing harmful effects. This topic brings attention to the evolving view of astrocytes as dynamic and influential players in CNS repair. By harnessing their regenerative potential, future therapeutic interventions may better support functional recovery after trauma or disease.

Keywords: proliferative reactive astrocytes, CNS injury, glial scar, neuroprotection, synaptic remodeling, astrogliosis

1. Introduction

Astrocytes, long overshadowed by neurons in the study of brain function, have undergone a dramatic reevaluation in recent decades. Traditionally viewed as passive scaffolding or homeostatic regulators within the central nervous system (CNS), astrocytes are now recognized as essential and highly dynamic participants in both health and disease [1]. This conceptual shift has brought attention to the diverse roles astrocytes play in synaptic transmission, metabolic support, blood-brain barrier (BBB) maintenance, and immune responses. Among the most striking demonstrations of their functional plasticity is the transformation of astrocytes into reactive phenotypes following CNS injury or disease [2].

Reactive astrogliosis is a complex and graded process by which astrocytes respond to various forms of CNS insult, ranging from trauma and ischemia to neurodegenerative disease and infection [3]. One significant and particularly compelling subtype of reactive astrocytes is the proliferative reactive astrocyte [4]. These cells emerge in response to severe or chronic injury and are characterized by a marked increase in mitotic activity, hypertrophy, and upregulation of glial fibrillary acidic protein (GFAP) and other intermediate filaments. While this proliferative response was once viewed predominantly as pathological, primarily for its role in glial scar formation and inhibition of axonal regeneration, it is now understood to be far more nuanced [5]. Proliferative reactive astrocytes occupy a dual role within the injured CNS. On one hand, they are involved in forming a dense glial barrier that contains inflammation and isolates damaged tissue. On the other hand, they participate actively in tissue repair processes, including restoration of the BBB, modulation of local inflammation, synaptic remodeling, and even the support of endogenous neurogenesis [6]. These astrocytes may therefore be seen not merely as scar-forming entities, but as context-sensitive regulators of CNS healing, capable of both promoting and impeding recovery depending on their activation state and the microenvironmental cues they receive [3, 7]. This duality has catalyzed a new wave of research focused on delineating the molecular signatures and functional heterogeneity of proliferative reactive astrocytes. Advances in single-cell RNA sequencing, lineage tracing, and in vivo imaging have begun to unravel the transcriptional diversity of reactive astrocytes, revealing that proliferation is not a uniform process but rather a specialized program orchestrated in a region- and time-dependent manner [8]. Specific signaling pathways, such as those involving STAT3, NF-κB, Notch, and Hippo-Yes-associated protein (YAP), have been implicated in governing the switch from quiescent to proliferative states, influencing not only the degree of astrogliosis but also its functional outcomes [9, 10].

A critical area of investigation concerns how these proliferative astrocytes interact with other CNS cells, including microglia, neurons, oligodendrocyte precursor cells (OPCs), and endothelial cells. The interplay between astrocytes and microglia, for instance, is essential for coordinating inflammatory responses and shaping the glial scar [11]. Proliferative astrocytes can secrete cytokines, chemokines, and extracellular matrix (ECM) molecules that modulate microglial activity and influence neuroimmune signaling [12, 13]. Their crosstalk with neurons is equally vital; astrocytes can stabilize synaptic circuits or prune dysfunctional synapses depending on the local injury context. Additionally, they provide metabolic and trophic support to neural progenitors, suggesting a role in facilitating limited neuroregeneration even in the adult CNS [14–16]. An emerging area of interest is the regional and temporal heterogeneity of proliferative astrocytes. Not all brain regions respond to injury with the same astrocytic profile. For example, cortical and hippocampal astrocytes may adopt distinct reactive phenotypes compared to those in the spinal cord or brainstem [17–19]. Moreover, the timing of proliferation, whether it occurs during the acute, subacute, or chronic phase of injury, has significant implications for therapeutic interventions [20–22]. Understanding how these differences manifest at molecular and functional levels could lead to more targeted and effective strategies for modulating astrocyte behavior in disease.

While much attention has been given to the maladaptive consequences of reactive astrogliosis, especially in the context of chronic inflammation and glial scarring, the therapeutic potential of proliferative reactive astrocytes is increasingly recognized. Efforts to manipulate astrocyte proliferation pharmacologically or genetically, either to enhance their reparative functions or mitigate their inhibitory effects, are gaining momentum. Some studies have explored ways to reprogram reactive astrocytes into neuroblasts or support their conversion into neurons in situ [23, 24]. Others focus on selectively inhibiting astrocytic signals that impede axonal regeneration while preserving their neuroprotective properties [25–27]. Despite these advances, several questions remain unanswered: What intrinsic and extrinsic factors determine whether a proliferative astrocyte will support regeneration or contribute to scar formation? Can the proliferative state be harnessed therapeutically without triggering tumorigenesis or other adverse effects? To what extent do age, sex, and genetic background influence the proliferative response? Addressing these questions requires a multidisciplinary approach that integrates molecular biology, systems neuroscience, neuroimmunology, and clinical pathology.

In this chapter, we aim to provide a comprehensive overview of proliferative reactive astrocytes in the CNS. The discussion is organized into several key thematic sections. First, we explore the molecular signatures that define these astrocytes, with an emphasis on transcriptional regulation, signaling pathways, and cell-cycle dynamics. Next, we examine their roles in inflammation, scar formation, and tissue repair, highlighting the balance between protective and detrimental outcomes. We then turn to the interactions between proliferative astrocytes and other CNS cell types, considering both direct cell-cell contact and paracrine signaling. The subsequent sections address their involvement in synaptic remodeling and neurogenesis, as well as the regional and temporal heterogeneity that shapes their functional profiles. Finally, we consider the therapeutic implications of modulating astrocyte proliferation and discuss future directions for research in this rapidly evolving field. Understanding the full repertoire of astrocyte responses to injury, particularly those involving proliferation, is crucial not only for basic neuroscience but also for the development of therapies aimed at treating CNS injuries and neurodegenerative diseases. Proliferative reactive astrocytes, once relegated to the margins of neuropathology, now stand at the forefront of CNS repair mechanisms. As our knowledge expands, the challenge will be to translate these insights into interventions that enhance the CNS's innate capacity for regeneration while minimizing maladaptive scarring. Here, we aim to provide a foundational understanding of the dynamic and multifaceted roles of proliferative reactive astrocytes within the injured central nervous system.

2. Molecular signatures of proliferative reactive astrocytes

Proliferative reactive astrocytes represent a distinct and highly regulated subset of astrocytes that emerge in response to CNS injury or disease. These cells are characterized by reentry into the cell cycle, altered transcriptional landscapes, and activation of signaling pathways that orchestrate both their proliferative and functional profiles. This section explores the intricate molecular architecture of proliferative reactive astrocytes, emphasizing transcriptional regulation, key signaling pathways, and the dynamics of cell-cycle reactivation (**Figure 1**).

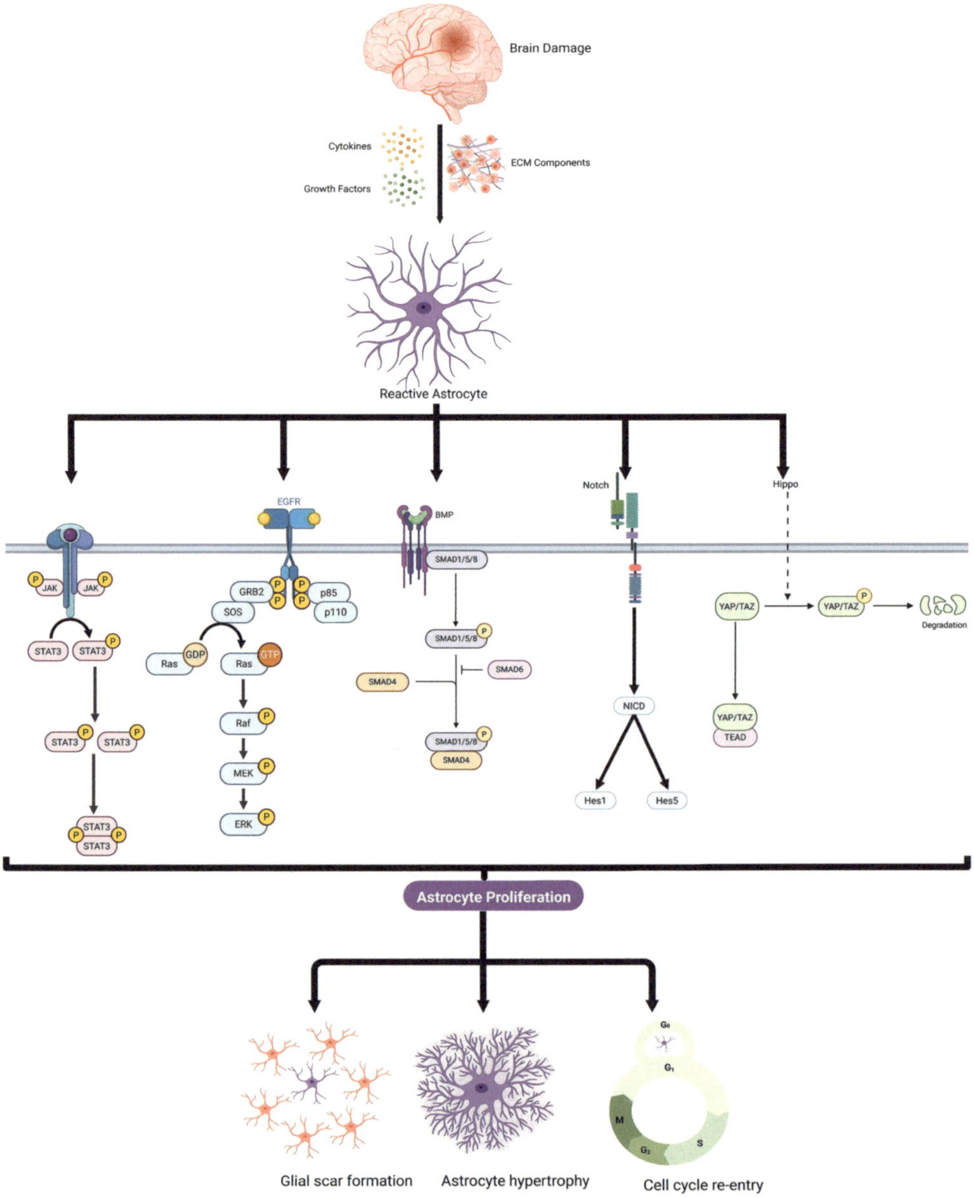

Figure 1.
Molecular signatures of proliferative reactive astrocytes. Proliferative reactive astrocytes emerge after CNS injury through coordinated transcriptional reprogramming, activation of key signaling pathways, and cell-cycle re-entry. Pathways including JAK/STAT, EGFR, Hippo-YAP, Notch, and BMP/TGF-β, regulate the transition from quiescence to proliferation. Downstream activation of cyclins, CDKs, and E2F enables mitotic reactivation, linking extracellular cues to functional outcomes in repair and scar formation.

2.1 Transcriptional reprogramming in reactive proliferation

One of the most defining features of proliferative reactive astrocytes is their robust transcriptional reprogramming in response to CNS injury. Upon activation, astrocytes shift from a quiescent, homeostatic state to a reactive phenotype, marked by the upregulation of cytoskeletal proteins such as GFAP, vimentin, and nestin [28–30]. However, proliferation involves an additional layer of transcriptional complexity. Key transcription factors orchestrate the gene expression programs that allow astrocytes to overcome mitotic quiescence and engage in cell division. Among the most well-characterized regulators is signal transducer and activator of transcription 3 (STAT3). STAT3 is rapidly activated following injury and drives the expression of genes involved in cytoskeletal remodeling, proliferation, and survival. Conditional deletion of STAT3 in astrocytes impairs their proliferation and alters the formation of the glial scar, demonstrating its essential role in reactive astrogliosis [31]. Another important transcription factor is nuclear factor kappa B (NF-κB), which mediates inflammatory signaling and cell survival. Activation of NF-κB in reactive astrocytes leads to the production of cytokines such as interleukin-1β (IL-1β) and tumor necrosis factor-alpha (TNF-α), which in turn can create a feedback loop promoting further astrocyte proliferation and glial scarring. Additional transcriptional regulators, such as Sox9, Olig2, and c-Myc, also contribute to the proliferative phenotype. Sox9, for instance, is required for maintaining astrocyte identity and promoting proliferation during injury response [31–34]. c-Myc, a well-known proto-oncogene, is transiently upregulated and contributes to cell-cycle entry, although its overexpression must be tightly controlled to prevent oncogenic transformation [34].

2.2 Key signaling pathways driving astrocyte proliferation

Astrocyte proliferation is not solely governed by intrinsic transcription factors; it is also shaped by the extracellular environment via several conserved signaling pathways. Among these, the JAK/STAT, EGFR, Hippo-YAP, Notch, and BMP/TGF-β pathways are of central importance. The JAK/STAT pathway, particularly involving STAT3 as discussed, is activated by cytokines such as IL-6 and leukemia inhibitory factor (LIF), both of which are upregulated in the injured CNS. This pathway not only supports proliferation but also contributes to the protective and reparative aspects of reactive astrocytes [35]. Epidermal growth factor receptor (EGFR) signaling is another driver of astrocyte proliferation. EGFR ligands such as EGF and TGF-α are upregulated in response to injury and promote mitogenic activity through downstream effectors like ERK and PI3K/AKT. EGFR activation can also synergize with STAT3 signaling, enhancing astrocyte expansion and contributing to the spatial organization of the glial scar [36, 37]. The Hippo-YAP signaling pathway is emerging as a key regulator of astrocyte proliferation and reactivity. Under normal conditions, Hippo signaling restrains YAP activity, keeping astrocytes in a nonproliferative state [38]. Following injury, inhibition of Hippo kinases allows YAP to translocate into the nucleus, where it partners with TEAD transcription factors to drive genes involved in proliferation and tissue remodeling [39]. Notch signaling plays a dual role in astrocyte biology: it maintains astrocyte identity during development and, in the adult CNS, contributes to injury-induced proliferation. Notch receptor activation by ligands such as Jagged1 triggers the release of the Notch intracellular domain (NICD), which enters the nucleus and alters gene expression, often in concert with STAT3 and NF-κB [40–42]. Finally, the BMP/TGF-β pathway regulates the balance between astrocyte proliferation and differentiation. While TGF-β can promote scar formation and astrocyte reactivity, it often acts in a context-dependent manner, sometimes limiting proliferation while promoting ECM deposition [43].

2.3 Cell-cycle dynamics and mitotic reactivation

The reactivation of the cell cycle in postmitotic astrocytes is a tightly regulated process. In their resting state, astrocytes are generally maintained in the G0 phase [44]. Injury-associated cues initiate reentry into the cell cycle, typically involving progression through G1/S and G2/M checkpoints. This process is mediated by a surge in cyclin expression, especially cyclin D1 and cyclin A2, and activation of cyclin-dependent kinases (CDKs), such as CDK4/6 and CDK2. These kinases phosphorylate retinoblastoma protein (Rb), releasing E2F transcription factors that drive the expression of S-phase genes [45]. Simultaneously, inhibitory molecules, such as $p27^{Kip1}$ are downregulated, removing brakes on cell-cycle progression [46]. Interestingly, not all reactive astrocytes enter mitosis; many may undergo endoreplication or partial cell-cycle activation without completing division, suggesting heterogeneity in proliferative potential even within the reactive population [47]. Astrocyte proliferation is typically transient and localized, with peak mitotic activity occurring within the first several days postinjury. However, chronic injury or degenerative diseases can maintain or reinitiate proliferation, often in maladaptive ways that promote scar maturation or ongoing inflammation [48].

3. Roles of proliferative reactive astrocytes in inflammation, scar formation, and tissue repair

Astrocytes are central players in the brain's response to injury, and their shift into a reactive state is a hallmark of CNS pathology. Among the various reactive states, proliferative reactive astrocytes form a particularly important subset due to their active roles in inflammation, glial scar formation, and the orchestration of tissue repair [49]. Their functions, however, are not strictly beneficial or harmful. Instead, they operate within a delicate balance, wherein their actions can either promote recovery or exacerbate damage, depending on the timing, severity, and nature of the insult. This section examines how proliferative astrocytes contribute to neuroinflammation, structural containment through scarring, and reparative processes, with special focus on how these outcomes are influenced by the cellular and molecular context (**Figure 2**).

3.1 Proliferative astrocytes in neuroinflammation

In response to CNS injury, whether due to trauma, ischemia, infection, or neurodegenerative disease, astrocytes become one of the first responders. This response includes morphological changes, upregulation of intermediate filaments like GFAP and vimentin, and, in more severe cases, entry into the cell cycle and proliferation.

Proliferative reactive astrocytes are actively involved in shaping the inflammatory environment. They release a range of cytokines and chemokines, including interleukin-6 (IL-6), TNF-α, IL-1β, CXCL10, and CCL2, which recruit and modulate the activity of immune cells such as microglia, monocytes, and T cells [50–54]. They also express major histocompatibility complex (MHC) molecules under certain conditions, enabling them to participate in antigen presentation and immune regulation [55]. This inflammatory role is context-dependent. In the early

DOI: http://dx.doi.org/10.5772/intechopen.1013131

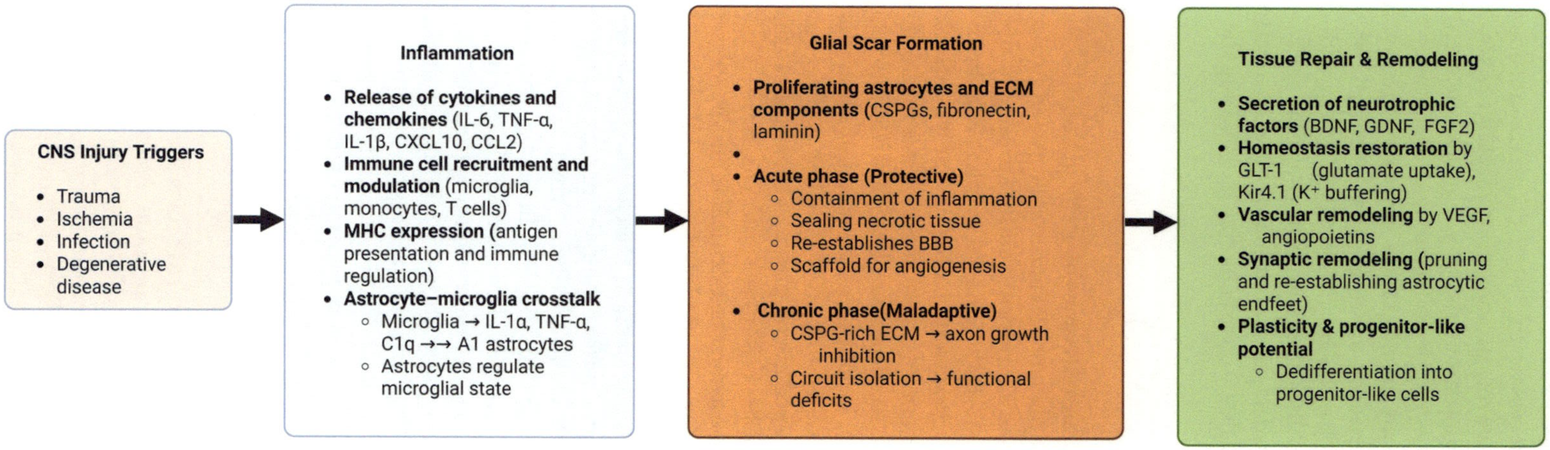

Figure 2.
Roles of proliferative reactive astrocytes in CNS injury. Proliferative reactive astrocytes orchestrate inflammation, scar formation, and tissue repair after injury. In the acute phase, they promote immune coordination, blood–brain barrier restoration, and neurotrophic support, whereas in the chronic phase, persistent proliferation contributes to maladaptive scarring, inhibitory extracellular matrix deposition, and prolonged inflammation. The balance between these protective and detrimental roles determines whether astrocyte proliferation supports recovery or exacerbates pathology..

phases of injury, astrocyte-derived cytokines help orchestrate innate and adaptive immune responses that are necessary for debris clearance, antimicrobial defense, and containment of damage. However, prolonged or excessive activation of astrocytes can perpetuate chronic inflammation, creating a hostile microenvironment that impedes regeneration, alters synaptic function, and contributes to secondary neuronal loss [56]. Additionally, proliferative astrocytes are involved in crosstalk with microglia, the brain's resident immune cells. This interaction is bidirectional: microglia-derived signals such as IL-1α, TNF-α, and C1q can induce astrocytes into a neurotoxic A1 phenotype, while astrocytes, in turn, influence microglial activation states [56]. The balance between pro-inflammatory and antiinflammatory signaling in this astrocyte-microglia dialogue is crucial for determining the overall outcome of the inflammatory response.

3.2 Glial scar formation: A double-edged sword

One of the most recognizable outcomes of astrocyte proliferation is the formation of the glial scar, a dense, multilayered structure composed primarily of astrocytes, along with ECM molecules like chondroitin sulfate proteoglycans (CSPGs), fibronectin, and laminin [26, 57–60]. The glial scar has long been viewed as a barrier to axonal regeneration, and historically, its formation was associated with poor functional recovery. However, more recent research has revealed that scar formation is not inherently detrimental. In the acute phase of CNS injury, the glial scar plays essential protective roles [61]. It contains the spread of inflammation and cytotoxic molecules, seals off necrotic tissue to prevent further tissue degradation, reestablishes the BBB in damaged areas, provides a scaffold for revascularization, and limits infiltration of peripheral immune cells [62, 63].

The proliferative aspect of astrocytes is critical in this process. Cell division allows astrocytes to populate the lesion site, replace lost astroglial support, and organize into a structurally coherent barrier. These functions are crucial in minimizing secondary injury [15, 64]. Nevertheless, in the chronic phase, the glial scar can become maladaptive. Astrocytes within the mature scar express high levels of inhibitory ECM molecules, particularly CSPGs, which actively repel axonal growth and hinder synaptic reconnection [61, 65]. Additionally, persistent scar formation can contribute to the isolation of neural circuits, leading to functional deficits, particularly in spinal cord injury and demyelinating diseases like multiple sclerosis. The degree and timing of astrocyte proliferation influence the nature of the scar [20–22]. Overactive proliferation can lead to excessive scarring and ECM deposition, while insufficient proliferation may fail to contain inflammation, resulting in tissue degradation [66–68]. Thus, fine-tuned regulation of astrocyte proliferation is essential to achieve a beneficial balance.

3.3 Contributions to tissue repair and remodeling

Beyond their role in containment and scar formation, proliferative reactive astrocytes contribute in profound ways to tissue repair and regenerative support. A major aspect of this contribution lies in their ability to secrete a wide array of neurotrophic factors, including brain-derived neurotrophic factor (BDNF), glial cell-derived neurotrophic factor (GDNF), and fibroblast growth factor 2 (FGF2). These molecules support neuronal survival, stimulate axonal sprouting, and promote synaptic plasticity, thereby establishing a permissive environment for functional recovery [69–71]. At the same time, astrocytes actively restore neurochemical and ionic homeostasis. By upregulating glutamate transporters such as GLT-1 and potassium channels like Kir4.1, they regulate excitatory neurotransmission and prevent excitotoxicity, which is particularly damaging in the aftermath of CNS injury [72–75]. Parallel to these functions, astrocytes also play an essential role in vascular remodeling. Through the release of pro-angiogenic molecules, including vascular endothelial growth factor (VEGF) and angiopoietins, they stimulate angiogenesis, thereby ensuring an adequate delivery of oxygen and nutrients to regenerating tissue [76–79]. At the synaptic level, reactive astrocytes take on a remodeling function, pruning damaged or dysfunctional synapses while reestablishing astrocytic endfeet at synaptic terminals, a process that helps to stabilize communication between neurons and restore local circuit integrity [14, 80].

Emerging evidence further suggests that proliferative astrocytes possess a degree of cellular plasticity that extends beyond supportive roles. In certain experimental models of injury, subpopulations of reactive astrocytes have demonstrated the ability to de-differentiate into progenitor-like states, adopting phenotypes reminiscent of neural stem or progenitor cells [81]. These cells exhibit the potential to generate new neurons or glial cells, highlighting a latent regenerative capacity within the astrocyte population. Although this phenomenon remains limited in mammals compared to highly regenerative species such as zebrafish, it underscores the versatility of astrocytes in orchestrating tissue repair [82, 83]. This capacity for cellular reprogramming has fueled growing interest in therapeutic strategies aimed at harnessing astrocytic plasticity, either through genetic reprogramming or pharmacological modulation, to promote neurogenesis and structural repair in the injured brain. Taken together, these observations reveal that reactive astrocytes are not simply barriers to regeneration; rather, they function as active, multifaceted participants in tissue remodeling, circuit stabilization, and regenerative support, making them central players in the complex choreography of recovery following CNS damage.

3.4 Striking the right balance

The dichotomous roles of proliferative reactive astrocytes, acting as both protectors and potential impediments, highlight the importance of context when evaluating their contributions to CNS pathology and repair. In the acute phases of injury, astrocytic proliferation and the upregulation of reactive signaling pathways are often protective, containing tissue damage, stabilizing the BBB, and limiting the spread of inflammation. Their ability to secrete neurotrophic and angiogenic factors at this stage helps sustain neuronal survival and initiate vascular and synaptic remodeling [6, 84]. However, if proliferation becomes excessive or persists into chronic stages, the same astrocytic responses can become maladaptive. Dense glial scar formation, deposition of axon-repelling ECM components, and the release of pro-inflammatory mediators can all interfere with long-term recovery by inhibiting axonal regrowth and prolonging neuroinflammation [29, 84]. Thus, the astrocytic response must be understood as temporally dynamic, with outcomes that are beneficial in the early stages of injury but potentially detrimental if left unchecked during chronic disease or the later phases of tissue remodeling [85].

Recognizing this duality, therapeutic approaches are increasingly aimed at recalibrating astrocytic behavior rather than suppressing their reactivity outright. Strategies under investigation include reprogramming reactive astrocytes into phenotypes that favor neuroprotection and regeneration [86–89], inhibiting the synthesis of inhibitory ECM molecules such as CSPGs, and even directing astrocytes toward neurogenic fates through transcriptional or pharmacological interventions [90, 91]. The challenge lies in identifying and manipulating the molecular switches, such as STAT3, NFκB, and Notch signaling pathways, that dictate whether reactive astrocytes adopt beneficial or inhibitory roles [33, 35, 86, 92–94]. As our understanding of these mechanisms deepens, the possibility of reshaping astrocytic plasticity for therapeutic gain becomes increasingly tangible. Proliferative reactive astrocytes should therefore not be viewed as passive responders but as active orchestrators of CNS repair, whose functions in inflammation, scar formation, and tissue remodeling are intricately regulated by timing and context [95]. The future of astrocyte-targeted therapies will depend on striking the right balance: amplifying their protective functions in the acute setting while curbing their inhibitory features during chronic disease progression.

4. Interactions between proliferative astrocytes and other CNS cell types

The CNS is a highly interconnected environment, where cellular communication is essential for homeostasis, defense, and repair. Within this framework, proliferative reactive astrocytes emerge as crucial players following injury or disease. Their interactions with neighboring CNS cells, such as neurons, microglia, oligodendrocyte lineage cells, endothelial cells, and neural stem or progenitor cells, are governed by a combination of direct physical contact and paracrine signaling, both of which modulate injury responses and shape long-term recovery outcomes (**Figure 3**).

4.1 Astrocyte-microglia interactions

Among the most extensively studied interactions are those between reactive astrocytes and microglia, the resident immune cells of the central nervous system. Microglia and astrocytes engage in a bidirectional communication loop, particularly during the acute and subacute phases of injury. Following CNS damage, activated microglia release a broad spectrum of cytokines, such as interleukin-1 beta, tumor necrosis factor-alpha, and interleukin-6 [96, 97]. These cytokines activate intracellular cascades in astrocytes, notably the STAT3 and NF-kappa B pathways, which amplify astrocyte reactivity, drive proliferation, and induce the expression of GFAP and ECM molecules, including CSPGs [9, 35, 41, 98].

Proliferative astrocytes, in turn, release mediators such as transforming growth factor beta, interleukin-10, and lipocalin-2 [99–101]. These molecules modulate the microglial phenotype by promoting a transition from pro-inflammatory to reparative states, characterized by enhanced phagocytic activity and the production of neurotrophic factors. Astrocytes also exert control through direct contact, utilizing cell surface ligands such as CD200 and CX3CL1, which engage microglial receptors CD200R and CX3CR1 and restrict excessive microglial activation [102–105]. Furthermore, astrocyte-derived ATP and glutamate further influence

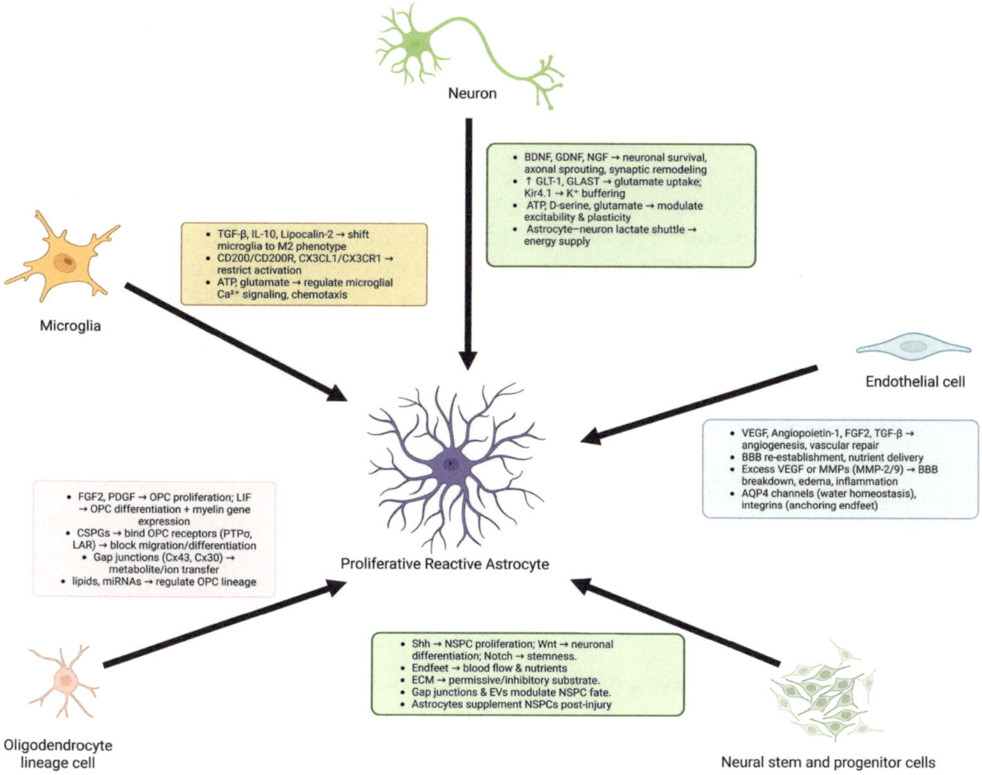

Figure 3.
Proliferative reactive astrocytes activated after CNS injury coordinate bidirectional interactions with surrounding cells. They modulate microglia via cytokines and anti-inflammatory signals, support neurons through trophic factors, neurotransmitter homeostasis, and metabolic coupling, influence oligodendrocytes/OPCs via growth factors, gap junctions, and ECM cues, regulate endothelial cells to promote angiogenesis and BBB repair, and control NSPCs through Shh, Wnt, Notch, and niche remodeling.

microglial calcium signaling and chemotactic behavior, adding additional layers of regulation [106, 107].

Persistent stimulation of these pathways can alter their functional outcomes. For example, sustained STAT3 signaling in astrocytes promotes prolonged proliferation and glial scar stabilization, while chronic microglial exposure to astrocyte-derived lipocalin-2 can reinforce pro-inflammatory signaling. These context-dependent dynamics highlight the complexity of astrocyte-microglia interactions during CNS injury, where the same molecular mediators may contribute to neuroprotection, repair, or pathological remodeling depending on timing, intensity, and cellular state [98, 100, 101].

4.2 Astrocyte-neuron crosstalk

Proliferative astrocytes maintain dynamic interactions with neurons that regulate both survival and functional recovery after injury. Reactive astrocytes secrete neurotrophic factors such as brain-derived neurotrophic factor, glial cell line-derived neurotrophic factor, and nerve growth factor, which enhance neuronal survival, support axonal sprouting, and facilitate synaptic remodeling [70, 108, 109]. In parallel, they control extracellular excitatory signaling by upregulating glutamate transporters GLT-1 and GLAST, thereby maintaining glutamate homeostasis and limiting excitotoxicity, a major contributor to delayed neuronal death in injured tissue [110–112].

Structural communication occurs through the tripartite synapse, in which astrocytic processes surround neuronal synaptic terminals. Even when reactive astrocytes undergo morphological changes during proliferation, they often preserve their capacity to modulate synaptic function [113, 114]. This regulation is achieved not only by buffering ions and neurotransmitters but also by releasing gliotransmitters such as ATP, D-serine, and glutamate, which act on pre and postsynaptic receptors to influence excitability and plasticity [115]. Calcium-dependent signaling within astrocytic endfeet is particularly important for coordinating this release and synchronizing neuronal network activity [116, 117]. Astrocytes additionally contribute to neuronal metabolic support by supplying lactate through the astrocyte-neuron lactate shuttle, which fuels axonal activity during periods of high energy demand [118–120]. They also regulate extracellular potassium concentrations via inward-rectifying potassium channels, helping stabilize neuronal firing patterns in the perilesional environment [121, 122]. These multilevel interactions integrate trophic support, metabolic coupling, and synaptic modulation, positioning proliferative astrocytes as active participants in the regulation of neuronal viability and circuit reorganization following CNS injury.

4.3 Astrocyte-oligodendrocyte lineage interactions

The relationship between reactive astrocytes and oligodendrocyte progenitor cells is a central determinant of remyelination after CNS injury. Astrocytes secrete a range of trophic and regulatory factors that influence OPC behavior. FGF 2 and platelet-derived growth factor act as potent mitogens that stimulate OPC proliferation and recruitment to demyelinated regions [123]. LIF promotes differentiation of OPCs into mature oligodendrocytes and enhances the expression of myelin basic protein and proteolipid protein, which are essential for myelin sheath formation [124]. In contrast, reactive astrocytes also produce ECM molecules such as CSPGs, which interact with OPC receptors, including protein tyrosine phosphatase sigma and leukocyte common antigen-related phosphatase, leading to cytoskeletal rearrangements that restrict migration and delay differentiation [125–127].

In addition to paracrine signaling, astrocytes engage in direct communication with OPCs. Gap junctions containing connexin 43 and connexin 30 establish intercellular coupling that enables the transfer of ions, metabolites, and small signaling molecules, thereby supporting metabolic homeostasis during periods of repair [128–131]. Astrocytes can also release extracellular vesicles enriched in lipids and microRNAs that modulate OPC lineage progression, adding another layer of regulation to this crosstalk. Moreover, astrocytic regulation of extracellular potassium and glutamate concentrations indirectly influences OPC physiology, as these progenitors are highly sensitive to ionic and neurotransmitter fluctuations in the lesion microenvironment [132–134]. These diverse signaling modalities highlight the capacity of proliferative reactive astrocytes to either facilitate or impede the progression of OPCs toward myelinating oligodendrocytes, depending on the balance of supportive versus inhibitory cues present in the injured CNS [135].

4.4 Astrocyte-endothelial interactions and the neurovascular unit

Proliferative reactive astrocytes play a crucial role in modulating cerebral vasculature through close interactions with endothelial cells, especially within the highly specialized neurovascular unit (NVU), which integrates neurons, astrocytes, endothelial cells, pericytes, and ECM components. The NVU ensures tight coupling between neuronal activity and vascular responses, and astrocytes are critical mediators of this cross-talk [136–138]. Astrocytic endfeet, which ensheath more than 90% of cerebral capillaries, form a dynamic interface between the brain parenchyma and blood vessels [139, 140]. Through this anatomical positioning, astrocytes contribute to both the maintenance and restoration of the BBB [141]. Following injury, reactive astrocytes undergo hypertrophy and upregulate the expression of several signaling molecules that influence endothelial physiology. For instance, they secrete angiogenic factors such as VEGF, angiopoietin-1, FGF2, and transforming growth factor-β (TGF-β), which promote endothelial cell survival, proliferation, and neovascularization. While moderate VEGF release is beneficial in restoring vascular supply, uncontrolled or excessive VEGF can compromise BBB integrity, leading to increased vascular permeability, leakage, and cerebral edema [142–145].

Astrocytes also maintain direct physical interactions with endothelial cells via adhesion molecules. Integrins facilitate structural anchoring of astrocytic endfeet to the vascular basement membrane, while aquaporin-4 (AQP4) channels regulate bidirectional water fluxes essential for edema clearance and homeostatic balance. Alterations in AQP4 localization or function are frequently observed in traumatic brain injury, stroke, and neurodegenerative disorders, highlighting its importance in BBB stability [139–141, 146, 147].

Another layer of regulation is mediated by astrocyte-derived matrix metalloproteinases (MMPs), particularly MMP-2 and MMP-9. These proteolytic enzymes remodel the ECM surrounding cerebral vessels, thereby facilitating angiogenesis and vascular repair. However, excessive or unregulated MMP activity may exacerbate BBB breakdown and inflammation by degrading tight junction proteins such as claudin-5, occludin, and ZO-1 [148]. Thus, the balance between constructive ECM remodeling and destructive barrier disruption is tightly governed by astrocyte–endothelial interactions. Collectively, these processes underscore the dual role of astrocytes in vascular pathology and repair. On one hand, they support angiogenesis, nutrient delivery, and BBB restoration; on the other, dysregulated astrocytic signaling may worsen vascular leakage and neuroinflammation. Understanding the fine balance of astrocyte–endothelial communication within the NVU is therefore essential for developing therapeutic strategies aimed at preserving BBB integrity and optimizing vascular recovery after CNS injury.

4.5 Astrocyte-neural stem/progenitor cell communication

In neurogenic regions such as the subventricular zone (SVZ) and the hippocampal dentate gyrus, reactive astrocytes play a central role in shaping the activity of neural stem and progenitor cells (NSPCs). They secrete a diverse repertoire of signaling molecules, including Sonic hedgehog (Shh), Wnt proteins, and Notch ligands, each of which exerts distinct effects on NSPC regulation. Shh signaling is closely associated with the maintenance of NSPC proliferation and the expansion of the progenitor pool following injury. Wnt ligands generally act to promote neuronal differentiation and synaptic integration, although their effects can vary with developmental stage and cellular context. Notch signaling, in contrast, tends to preserve stemness by inhibiting premature differentiation, thereby ensuring a balance between self-renewal and lineage commitment [149–153]. In this way, astrocytes act as dynamic modulators of NSPC behavior, fine-tuning proliferation and differentiation in response to local conditions.

Beyond soluble signaling, astrocytes influence NSPCs through structural and metabolic support. Their endfeet form intimate contacts with the vasculature, allowing astrocytes to regulate local blood flow, nutrient exchange, and metabolic coupling between the niche and neural progenitors. Reactive astrocytes also remodel the ECM, depositing or degrading molecules such as laminins and CSPGs, which can either create permissive substrates for neurogenesis or establish inhibitory barriers that restrict progenitor migration and differentiation. These bidirectional interactions with the ECM further diversify the ways in which astrocytes control the neurogenic microenvironment [154–157]. A particularly interesting line of study suggests that astrocytes themselves may adopt progenitor-like features under certain pathological or experimentally manipulated conditions [81, 158, 159]. In some injury models, subsets of astrocytes begin to express neural stem cell markers, proliferate, and even generate neurons or oligodendrocytes. This phenomenon of transdifferentiation remains controversial, as lineage-tracing studies have yielded variable results, but it highlights the potential latent plasticity within mature astrocytes. Even if true transdifferentiation is rare, the capacity of astrocytes to revert to a progenitor-like state suggests that they may serve as a cellular reservoir for repair, complementing their role as niche regulators [158, 159]. Through this combination of soluble signaling, ECM remodeling, metabolic support, and potential lineage plasticity, reactive astrocytes exert multifaceted control over NSPC dynamics in neurogenic regions. Their influence is not uniform but varies with injury severity, timing, and molecular cues in the surrounding microenvironment, giving rise to outcomes that can either favor regeneration or limit repair.

5. Roles in synaptic remodeling, neurogenesis, and functional heterogeneity

5.1 The involvement of proliferative reactive astrocytes in synaptic remodeling

One of the most significant contributions of proliferative reactive astrocytes is their role in synaptic remodeling, which includes the modulation of synaptic structure, function, and connectivity. These functions are essential during CNS recovery, as they influence both the elimination of damaged synapses and the stabilization or formation of new connections. Even under homeostatic conditions, astrocytes are essential regulators of synaptic activity. They form tripartite synapses by extending their fine perisynaptic processes around synaptic junctions, enabling them to modulate neurotransmission, neurotransmitter uptake, and ionic balance [113, 114, 136, 160]. When these astrocytes adopt a reactive and proliferative phenotype following CNS injury, they undergo morphological transformations that allow them to dynamically interact with affected synapses. This remodeling is mediated through the reorganization of their cytoskeleton, involving the upregulation of proteins like GFAP, vimentin, and nestin, which support hypertrophy and process extension or retraction (**Figure 4**) [34, 97].

DOI: http://dx.doi.org/10.5772/intechopen.1013131

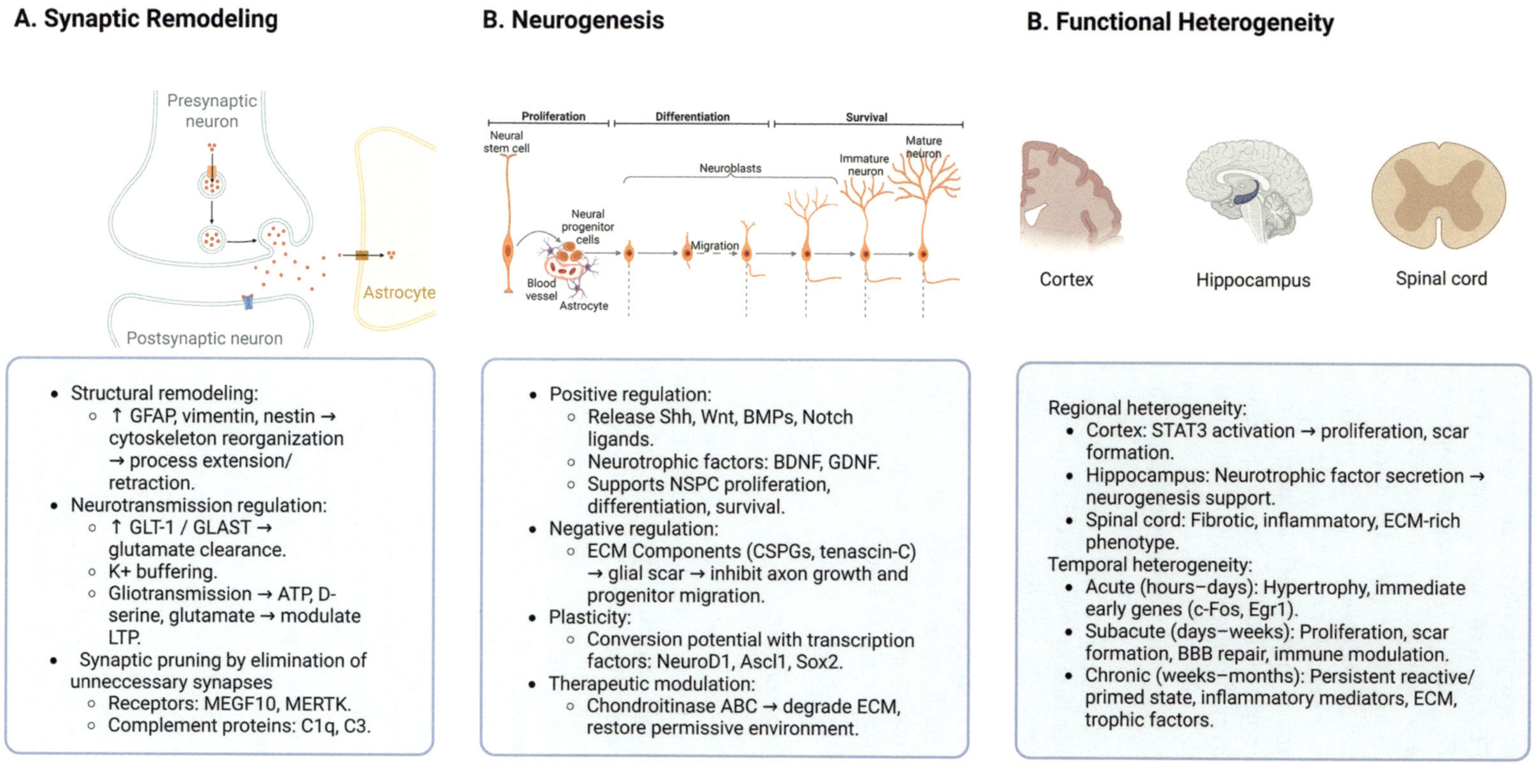

Figure 4.

Roles of Proliferative Reactive Astrocytes in Synaptic Remodeling, Neurogenesis, and Functional Heterogeneity. Proliferative reactive astrocytes modulate synaptic structure and function via tripartite synapses, cytoskeletal remodeling (GFAP, vimentin, nestin), neurotransmitter clearance (GLT-1/GLAST), K^+ buffering, gliotransmission, and synaptic pruning (MEGF10/MERTK, C1q/C3), influencing plasticity and cognitive outcomes. In neurogenic niches (SVZ, hippocampus), they support NSPC proliferation, differentiation, and survival through Shh, Wnt, BMPs, Notch ligands, and neurotrophic factors, while ECM components (CSPGs, tenascin-C) inhibit growth in non-neurogenic regions; astrocyte plasticity allows transcription factor-driven conversion and therapeutic ECM modulation. Functional heterogeneity is evident across regions (cortex, hippocampus, spinal cord) and time (acute → subacute → chronic), with dynamic shifts in proliferation, scar formation, immune modulation, trophic factor secretion, and epigenetic memory contributing to adaptive or maladaptive outcomes.

Beyond structural remodeling, proliferative reactive astrocytes exert regulatory control over synaptic transmission. One of their critical roles postinjury is glutamate clearance, achieved through the upregulation of transporters such as GLT-1 (EAAT2) and GLAST (EAAT1), which prevent excitotoxic damage caused by excessive glutamate accumulation. They also help maintain extracellular potassium balance by buffering ion concentrations during heightened neuronal activity [161]. Additionally, reactive astrocytes engage in gliotransmission, releasing signaling molecules like ATP, D-serine, and glutamate, which influence synaptic efficacy and can alter plasticity mechanisms such as long-term potentiation (LTP) [162]. A less obvious but critical contribution of proliferative astrocytes to synaptic remodeling is their involvement in synaptic pruning. Through the expression of phagocytic receptors such as MEGF10 and MERTK, as well as the engagement of complement cascade proteins like C1q and C3, astrocytes participate in tagging and eliminating dysfunctional or unnecessary synapses [163, 164]. This role is especially important during the subacute phase of injury, when neuronal circuits undergo active reorganization. While this pruning is often beneficial for recovery, aberrant or excessive astrocytic pruning has been linked to cognitive decline and synaptic loss in conditions like Alzheimer's disease [165–167]. Altogether, the contributions of proliferative reactive astrocytes to synaptic remodeling are multitiered, encompassing structural support, modulation of neurotransmission, synaptic pruning, and signaling cross-talk with neurons. These roles are essential for both immediate neuroprotection and long-term reorganization of neural networks following CNS injury.

5.2 Their roles in neurogenesis

Beyond their role at synapses, proliferative reactive astrocytes play a crucial part in modulating adult neurogenesis, especially in the two primary neurogenic niches of the adult brain: the SVZ and the hippocampal dentate gyrus [15, 168]. In these regions, astrocytes are integral to the regulation of NSPCs, influencing their proliferation, differentiation, and integration into existing neural circuits. After CNS injury, reactive astrocytes release a host of signaling molecules that shape the local neurogenic environment [169]. These include Shh, Wnt proteins, bone morphogenetic proteins (BMPs), Notch ligands, and a range of cytokines and growth factors [170]. Depending on the phase of injury and the surrounding milieu, these factors may either suppress or enhance neurogenesis. For example, during the acute phase of injury, astrocytes may secrete signals that inhibit progenitor proliferation, likely as a protective mechanism to prevent disorganized growth in a hostile, inflamed environment [48, 171]. However, during the recovery phase, they may switch to releasing neurotrophic factors like BDNF and GDNF, which promote the survival, maturation, and integration of newborn neurons. In experimental models, forced expression of transcription factors such as NeuroD1, Ascl1, or Sox2 can induce the conversion of reactive astrocytes into functional neurons, both in vitro and in vivo [108, 172, 173]. While the natural occurrence of such transdifferentiation in unmanipulated settings is still under debate, the concept suggests that proliferative astrocytes retain a degree of latent plasticity that could be therapeutically harnessed [158]. However, it is important to recognize that outside the SVZ and hippocampus, the role of reactive astrocytes in neurogenesis becomes more complex and often more inhibitory. In nonneurogenic regions such as the cortex or spinal cord, proliferative astrocytes tend to produce ECM components, like CSPGs and tenascin-C, which form part of the glial scar and actively inhibit axonal growth and progenitor cell migration [174, 175]. These molecules create a nonpermissive environment for neurogenesis. Yet, studies using enzymes like chondroitinase ABC have demonstrated that degrading these ECM components can enhance neurogenic potential and promote neural repair, indicating that astrocyte-mediated inhibition is not irreversible [176]. In sum, the influence of proliferative reactive astrocytes on neurogenesis is multifactorial and context-dependent. In neurogenic zones, they can provide trophic support and signaling cues that enable regeneration. In nonneurogenic regions, they often construct inhibitory environments, though even these effects can be modulated with therapeutic intervention.

5.3 Regional and temporal heterogeneity that shape their functional profiles

One of the most critical aspects of proliferative reactive astrocyte biology is their heterogeneity, both regional and temporal, which profoundly influences their roles in synaptic remodeling, neurogenesis, and overall CNS recovery. Astrocytes are not a monolithic population; their functions are determined by developmental lineage, anatomical location, and external stimuli. Regionally, astrocytes display distinct molecular signatures and activation patterns [177, 178]. For instance, cortical astrocytes following ischemic stroke tend to exhibit strong STAT3 activation, leading to pronounced proliferation and scar formation. These cells typically express high levels of GFAP and ECM molecules that support glial barrier functions [35, 179]. Conversely, hippocampal astrocytes, especially those in the dentate gyrus, are more involved in modulating the neurogenic niche and secrete a broader array of neurotrophic factors. In the spinal cord, astrocytes are often more fibrotic and inhibitory, upregulating genes associated with inflammation and ECM remodeling. These regional distinctions are not merely academic; they have real functional implications for how the CNS heals or degenerates following insult [168, 180, 181]. Equally important is the temporal progression of astrocyte responses. The transformation of astrocytes into a reactive, proliferative state occurs in phases, each with distinct functional attributes. During the acute phase (hours to days postinjury), astrocytes become hypertrophic and begin expressing immediate early genes like c-Fos and Egr1. Some begin to proliferate in response to mitogenic cues such as EGF and FGF2, initiating the early stages of tissue stabilization and immune modulation [177, 182]. In the subacute phase (days to weeks), proliferative astrocytes actively contribute to glial scar formation, help restore BBB integrity, and shape the immune microenvironment. This period represents a therapeutic window where interventions might shift astrocyte behavior toward neuroprotection and plasticity rather than chronic inhibition [183]. Finally, during the chronic phase (weeks to months), astrocytes often adopt a more stabilized phenotype, although some may persist in a "primed" or partially reactive state. These astrocytes continue to influence CNS architecture through long-term secretion of inflammatory mediators, ECM components, or trophic factors [184]. Adding further complexity, there is growing evidence that reactive astrocytes can retain memory of prior insults. Epigenetic reprogramming and altered chromatin states can lead to a "trained" or "primed" astrocyte phenotype, particularly in the context of chronic neuroinflammation or repeated injuries [185]. These cells may respond more robustly or maladaptively to subsequent insults, contributing to disease progression or impaired recovery in conditions such as multiple sclerosis or traumatic brain injury [186]. Together, the regional and temporal heterogeneity of proliferative astrocytes reflects a highly adaptable system that responds to both the nature and timing of injury. These variations are crucial for determining whether astrocytes function primarily as protective, regenerative agents, or as obstacles to recovery.

6. Therapeutic implications of modulating astrocyte proliferation and future research directions

Astrocyte proliferation is a double-edged sword. On one hand, astrocytes that divide after injury contribute to glial scar formation, which acts as a barrier to further tissue damage, limits the spread of inflammation, and restores the BBB. These proliferating cells also help contain cytotoxic debris and promote local homeostasis. On the other hand, the dense scar matrix they contribute to, rich in ECM proteins like CSPGs, can inhibit axonal regeneration, cell migration, and synaptic reorganization, creating a nonpermissive environment for neuronal repair [6, 61, 65, 183, 187]. As such, the therapeutic potential of targeting proliferative astrocytes lies in achieving a delicate balance: restraining their inhibitory actions while enhancing their neuroprotective and regenerative capacities. One potential approach involves timing the modulation of astrocyte proliferation. Experimental models have shown that conditional ablation of proliferative astrocytes early after injury can worsen outcomes by exacerbating inflammation and neuronal loss [188]. Conversely, delaying inhibition of their proliferation until after the acute protective phase may reduce glial scarring and enhance axonal regrowth [189]. Such temporal selectivity could be achieved through small molecules or gene therapies that target key signaling pathways governing astrocyte proliferation, including JAK/STAT3, EGFR, Notch, and mTOR signaling. Modulating these pathways has already shown promise in preclinical studies, with some interventions leading to reduced gliosis, improved synaptic integration, and partial restoration of motor or cognitive function [190–193].

In parallel, the idea of reprogramming reactive astrocytes into neurons or oligodendrocyte progenitor-like cells has gained momentum. Several studies have demonstrated that, under certain conditions, astrocytes can be converted in situ into functional neurons [194–196]. This strategy holds promise for neurodegenerative diseases or injuries in nonneurogenic brain regions, where endogenous repair is limited. Importantly, since proliferative astrocytes are more plastic and transcriptionally active, they may represent an ideal starting population for such reprogramming efforts. However, challenges remain in controlling the efficiency, specificity, and safety of such conversions in vivo. Another therapeutic opportunity lies in fine-tuning the secretory profile of reactive astrocytes, many of which are influenced by their proliferative state. Proliferative astrocytes secrete a mix of pro- and antiinflammatory cytokines, trophic factors, and extracellular vesicles that influence the behavior of neurons, microglia, and oligodendrocyte lineage cells [197–199]. Interventions that bias this secretome toward a neuroprotective or regenerative phenotype could amplify the positive effects of astrocyte proliferation while minimizing harmful consequences. For instance, modulating astrocytic NF-κB or Nrf2 pathways has been shown to shift cytokine output and enhance neuronal survival in models of stroke and traumatic brain injury [200]. A growing interest has also emerged in the field of biomaterials and tissue engineering, where astrocyte biology is being integrated into the design of therapeutic scaffolds. Engineered hydrogels or injectable materials that interact with endogenous astrocytes, or even deliver proliferative astrocyte populations with tailored phenotypes, are being explored as means to support CNS regeneration. Such materials can be embedded with bioactive cues that influence astrocyte proliferation, differentiation, and scar formation [201, 202]. These strategies offer a platform to manipulate the injury environment locally, reducing the need for systemic drugs that carry broader side effects.

Despite these advances, several challenges continue to limit the clinical translation of astrocyte-targeted therapies. A major hurdle is the heterogeneity of reactive astrocytes, both across CNS regions and within a single injury context [3, 203]. Not all proliferative astrocytes are functionally equivalent, and broad manipulation risks unintended effects. For example, inhibiting proliferation in astrocytes that serve protective or neurogenic functions may impair recovery, while promoting proliferation in already fibrotic regions may worsen scarring. As such, future therapies must be highly specific, targeting particular subtypes, temporal windows, and anatomical sites [95]. Advances in single-cell RNA sequencing, spatial transcriptomics, and in vivo lineage tracing are beginning to reveal the diversity of astrocyte responses and could soon enable precision interventions [204].

Looking forward, several future research directions stand out as critical. First, there is a need to map the molecular identities of proliferative astrocyte subtypes across injury models and disease states. This could enable the development of markers for therapeutic targeting or cell sorting. Second, researchers must develop better tools for in vivo manipulation of astrocyte proliferation, ideally ones that allow reversible or graded control rather than binary on-and-off approaches. Third, it is essential to conduct more studies in large animal models or systems that more accurately reflect human CNS pathology, as most current insights derive from rodent models with limited translational potential. Another promising area lies in combination therapies, where modulation of astrocyte proliferation is paired with neurotrophic support, antiinflammatory treatment, or rehabilitation training to enhance recovery. The interplay between astrocytes and other glial cells, especially microglia and oligodendrocytes, is also ripe for investigation, as targeting astrocytes alone may be insufficient for full functional restoration. Finally, as personalized medicine continues to evolve, tailoring astrocyte-targeted therapies to individual injury profiles, genetic backgrounds, and disease progression stages will likely be necessary for optimal efficacy.

7. Conclusion

In a nutshell, the modulation of astrocyte proliferation holds substantial therapeutic promise for CNS injury and disease. These cells are not merely structural fillers but active agents of repair, inflammation, and plasticity. By harnessing their diverse capabilities, while mitigating their potential to impede regeneration, future therapies may achieve more robust and lasting neurological recovery. Continued investment in understanding their biology, heterogeneity, and interactions will be essential for turning this promise into clinical reality. Looking forward, the challenge will lie in developing strategies that can fine-tune astrocytic responses in a context-dependent manner, amplifying their protective and pro-regenerative functions while suppressing maladaptive processes such as glial scarring or excessive inflammation. Achieving this balance will likely require integrating molecular, genetic, and biomaterial approaches with advanced imaging and single-cell profiling techniques, enabling precise targeting of astrocyte subpopulations in both space and time. If successful, such efforts will not only open new therapeutic avenues for conditions ranging from traumatic brain and spinal cord injury to neurodegenerative disease but also reshape our broader understanding of CNS repair and resilience.

Conflict of Interest

The authors declare no conflicts of interest.

Acknowledgments

X.G. acknowledgs support from National Institutes of Health (NIH R56 NS129438, NS131465-01) and Falk Medical Research Trust. Really appreicate Anne Gowan for grammar and spelling check

The authorship criteria are listed in our Authorship Policy: https://www.intechopen.com/page/authorship-policy.

This section of your manuscript may also include funding information.

Author details

Lilesh Kumar Pradhan[1] and Xiang Gao[1*]
Spinal Cord and Brain Injury Research Group, Department of Neurological Surgery, Stark Neurosciences Research Institute, Indiana University School of Medicine, Indianapolis, USA

*Address all correspondence to: xiangao@iu.edu

References

[1] Sofroniew MV. Molecular dissection of reactive astrogliosis and glial scar formation. Trends in Neurosciences. 2009;**32**:638–647

[2] Verkhratsky A, Butt A, Li B, Illes P, Zorec R, Semyanov A, et al. Astrocytes in human central nervous system diseases: A frontier for new therapies. Signal Transduction and Targeted Therapy. 2023;**8**:396

[3] Escartin C, Galea E, Lakatos A, O'Callaghan JP, Petzold GC, Serrano-Pozo A, et al. Reactive astrocyte nomenclature, definitions, and future directions. Nature Neuroscience. 2021;**24**:312–325

[4] Yu GL, Zhang Y, Ning B. Reactive astrocytes in central nervous system injury: Subgroup and potential therapy. Frontiers in Cellular Neuroscience. 2021;**15**:792764

[5] Kumar A, Fontana IC, Nordberg A. Reactive astrogliosis: A friend or foe in the pathogenesis of Alzheimer's disease. Journal of Neurochemistry. 2023;**164**:309–324

[6] Zhou Y, Shao A, Yao Y, Tu S, Deng Y, Zhang J. Dual roles of astrocytes in plasticity and reconstruction after traumatic brain injury. Cell Communication and Signaling. 2020;**18**:62

[7] Pekny M, Pekna M. Reactive gliosis in the pathogenesis of CNS diseases. Biochimica Et Biophysica Acta (BBA) - Molecular Basis of Disease. 2016;**1862** (3):483–491. https://www.sciencedirect.com/science/article/pii/S0925443915003531 [Accessed: 2025-June-28]

[8] Gao MY, Wang JQ, He J, Gao R, Zhang Y, Li X. Single-Cell RNA-sequencing in astrocyte development, heterogeneity, and disease. Cellular and Molecular Neurobiology. 2023;**43**:3449–3464

[9] Tsuda M, Kohro Y, Yano T, Tsujikawa T, Kitano J, Tozaki-Saitoh H, et al. JAK-STAT3 pathway regulates spinal astrocyte proliferation and neuropathic pain maintenance in rats. Brain 2011;**134**:1127–1139

[10] Zhang H, Zhou Y, Cui B, Liu Z, Shen H. Novel insights into astrocyte-mediated signaling of proliferation, invasion and tumor immune microenvironment in glioblastoma. Biomedicine and Pharmacotherapy. 2020;**126**:110086

[11] Matejuk A, Ransohoff RM. Crosstalk between astrocytes and microglia: An overview. Frontiers in Immunology. 2020;**11**:1416

[12] Cekanaviciute E, Buckwalter MS. Astrocytes: Integrative Regulators of Neuroinflammation in stroke and other neurological diseases. Neurotherapeutics. 2016;**13**:685–701

[13] Wiese S, Karus M, Faissner A. Astrocytes as a source for extracellular matrix molecules and cytokines. Frontiers in Pharmacology. JUN; 2012. p. 3:120

[14] Lee HG, Wheeler MA, Quintana FJ. Function and therapeutic value of astrocytes in neurological diseases. Nature Reviews Drug Discovery. 2022;**21**:339–358

[15] Chiareli RA, Carvalho GA, Marques BL, Mota LS, Oliveira-Lima OC, Gomes RM, et al. The role of astrocytes in the Neurorepair process. Frontiers in Cell and Developmental Biology. 2021;**9**:665795

[16] Lee SY, Chung WS. Astrocytic crosstalk with brain and immune cells in healthy and diseased conditions. Current Opinion in Neurobiology. 2024;**84**:102840

[17] White RE, McTigue DM, Jakeman LB.Regional heterogeneity in astrocyte responses following contusive spinal cord injury in mice. Journal of Comparative Neurology. 2010;**518**(8):1370–1390

[18] Yoon H, Walters G, Paulsen AR, Scarisbrick IA.Astrocyte heterogeneity across the brain and spinal cord occurs developmentally, in adulthood and in response to demyelination. PLoS One. 2017;**12**(7):e0180697

[19] Duran RCD, Wang CY, Zheng H, Deneen B, Wu JQ. Brain region-specific gene signatures revealed by distinct astrocyte subpopulations unveil links to glioma and neurodegenerative diseases. eNeuro. 2019;**6**(2): DOI: 10.1523/ENEURO.0288-18.2019

[20] Collyer E, Blanco-Suarez E. Astrocytes in stroke-induced neurodegeneration: A timeline. Frontiers in Molecular Medicine. 2023;3:1240862

[21] Chen W, Su G, Chai M, An Y, Song J, Zhang Z. Astrogliosis and glial scar in ischemic stroke - focused on mechanism and treatment. Experimental Neurology. 2025;**385**:115131. https://www.sciencedirect.com/science/article/pii/S0014488624004576

[22] Michinaga S, Koyama Y. Pathophysiological responses and roles of astrocytes in traumatic brain injury. International Journal of Molecular Sciences. 2021;**22**:6418

[23] Torper O, Götz M. Brain repair from intrinsic cell sources: Turning reactive glia into neurons. Progress in Brain Research. 2017;**230**:69–97

[24] Huang L, Lai X, Liang X, Chen J, Yang Y, Xu W, et al. A promise for neuronal repair: Reprogramming astrocytes into neurons in vivo. Bioscience Reports. 2024;**44**: BSR20231717

[25] Wang C, Li L. The critical role of KLF4 in regulating the activation of A1/A2 reactive astrocytes following ischemic stroke. Journal of Neuroinflammation. 2023;**20**(1):44

[26] Quan L, Uyeda A, Manabe I, Muramatsu R.Astrocytic heterogeneous nuclear ribonucleoprotein U is involved in scar formation after spinal cord injury. Journal of Neuroinflammation. 2025;**22**(1):28

[27] Whiteman S, Askvig J. Astrocytic role of Thy-1 induced inhibition of axonal sprouting. Neural Regeneration Research. 2021;**16**:1192–1193

[28] Lazic A, Balint V, Ninkovic DS, Peric M, Stevanovic M. Reactive and Senescent Astroglial Phenotypes as Hallmarks of Brain Pathologies. International Journal of Molecular Sciences. 2022;**23**:4995

[29] Yuan Y, Liu H, Dai Z, He C, Qin S, Su Z.From Physiology to Pathology of Astrocytes: Highlighting Their Potential as Therapeutic Targets for CNS Injury. Neuroscience Bulletin. 2025;**41**(1):131–154

[30] Gabel S, Koncina E, Dorban G, Heurtaux T, Birck C, Glaab E, et al. Inflammation Promotes a Conversion of Astrocytes into Neural Progenitor Cells via NF-κB Activation. Molecular Neurobiology 2016;**53**:5041–5055

[31] Ageeva T, Rizvanov A, Mukhamedshina Y.NF-κB and JAK/STAT Signaling Pathways as Crucial Regulators of Neuroinflammation and Astrocyte Modulation in Spinal Cord Injury. Cells. 2024;**13**(7):581

[32] Buffo A, Vosko MR, Ertürk D, Hamann GF, Jucker M, Rowitch D, et al. Expression pattern of the transcription factor Olig2 in response to brain injuries: Implications for neuronal repair. Proceedings of the National Academy of Sciences 2005;**102**:18183–18188

[33] Brambilla R, Bracchi-Ricard V, Hu WH, Frydel B, Bramwell A, Karmally S, et al. Inhibition of astroglial nuclear factor κB reduces inflammation and improves functional recovery after spinal cord injury. The Journal of Experimental Medicine 2005;**202**:145–156

[34] Lassman AB, C DAI, Fuller GN, Vickers AJ, Holland EC.Overexpression of c-MYC promotes an undifferentiated phenotype in cultured astrocytes and allows elevated Ras and Akt signaling to induce gliomas from GFAP-expressing cells in mice. Neuron Glia Biology. 2004;**1**(2):157–163

[35] Herrmann JE, Imura T, Song B, Qi J, Ao Y, Nguyen TK, et al. STAT3 is a critical regulator of astrogliosis and scar formation after spinal cord injury. Journal of Neuroscience 2008;**28**:7231–7243

[36] Sheng QW, shi TD, bao GZ, Fang J, Zhang Q, Yu ZY, et al. Inhibition of EGFR/MAPK signaling reduces microglial inflammatory response and the associated secondary damage in rats after spinal cord injury. Journal of Neuroinflammation. 2012;**9.**

[37] Sriram K, Benkovic SA, Hebert MA, Miller DB, O'Callaghan JP. Induction of gp130-related cytokines and activation of JAK2/STAT3 pathway in astrocytes precedes up-regulation of glial fibrillary acidic protein in the 1-methyl-4-phenyl-1,2,3,6-tetrahydropyridine model of neurodegeneration: Key signaling pathway for astrogliosis in vivo? Journal of Biological Chemistry. 2004;**279**(19):19936–19947

[38] Huang Z, Wang Y, Hu G, Zhou J, Mei L, Xiong WC.YAP Is a Critical Inducer of SOCS3, Preventing Reactive Astrogliosis. Cerebral Cortex. 2016;**26**(5):2299–2310

[39] Zhang J, Xu X, Liu H, Jin L, Shen X, Xie C, et al. Astrocytic YAP prevents the demyelination through promoting expression of cholesterol synthesis genes in experimental autoimmune encephalomyelitis. Cell Death & Disease. 2021;**12**(10):907

[40] Marumo T, Takagi Y, Muraki K, Hashimoto N, Miyamoto S, Tanigaki K. Notch signaling regulates nucleocytoplasmic Olig2 translocation in reactive astrocytes differentiation after ischemic stroke. Neuroscience Research. 2013;**75**(3):204–209

[41] LeComte MD, Shimada IS, Sherwin C, Spees JL. Notch1-STAT3-ETBR signaling axis controls reactive astrocyte proliferation after brain injury. Proceedings of the National Academy of Sciences of the United States of America. 2015;**112**(28):8726–8731

[42] Acaz-Fonseca E, Ortiz-Rodriguez A, Azcoitia I, Garcia-Segura LM, Arevalo MA. Notch signaling in astrocytes mediates their morphological response to an inflammatory challenge. Cell Death Discovery. 2019;5(1):85

[43] Yang R, Zhang Y, Kang J, Zhang C, Ning B. Notch1–STAT3–ETBR signaling axis controls reactive astrocyte proliferation after brain injury. Proceedings of the National Academy of Sciences. 2024;**15**:8726–8731

[44] Urbán N, Blomfield IM, Guillemot F. Quiescence of Adult Mammalian Neural Stem Cells: A Highly Regulated Rest. Neuron. 2019;**104**(5):834–848. https://www.sciencedirect.com/science/article/pii/S0896627319308001#bib101

[45] Topacio BR, Zatulovskiy E, Cristea S, Xie S, Tambo CS, Rubin SM, et al. Cyclin D-Cdk4,6 Drives Cell-Cycle Progression via the Retinoblastoma Protein's C-Terminal Helix. Molecular Cell. 2019;**74**(4):758–770.e4. https://www.sciencedirect.com/science/article/pii/S1097276519302242

[46] Shirane M, Harumiya Y, Ishida N, Hirai A, Miyamoto C, Hatakeyama S, et al. Down-regulation of p27(Kip1) by two mechanisms, ubiquitin-mediated degradation and proteolytic processing. Journal of Biological Chemistry 1999;**274**:13886–13893

[47] Anderson MA, Ao Y, Sofroniew MV. Heterogeneity of reactive astrocytes. Neuroscience Letters. 2014;**565**:23–29

[48] Alhadidi QM, Bahader GA, Arvola O, Kitchen P, Shah ZA, Salman MM. Astrocytes in functional recovery following central nervous system injuries. The Journal of Physiology. 2024;**602**:3069–3096

[49] Bhatt M, Sharma M, Das B.The Role of Inflammatory Cascade and Reactive Astrogliosis in Glial Scar Formation Post-spinal Cord Injury. Cellular and Molecular Neurobiology. 2024;**44**(1):78

[50] HG L, JH L, Flausino LE, Quintana FJ. Neuroinflammation: An astrocyte perspective. Science Translational Medicine. 2023;**15**(721):eadi7828

[51] Brambilla R, Persaud T, Hu X, Karmally S, Shestopalov VI, Dvoriantchikova G, et al. Transgenic inhibition of astroglial NF-κB improves functional outcome in experimental autoimmune encephalomyelitis by suppressing chronic central nervous system inflammation. The Journal of Immunology 2009;**182**:2628–2640

[52] E MK, Ma JH, Guo F, Miers L, Lee E, Bannerman P, et al. Deletion of astroglial CXCL10 delays clinical onset but does not affect progressive axon loss in a murine autoimmune multiple sclerosis model. Journal of Neuroinflammation. 2014;**11**

[53] Kim RY, Hoffman AS, Itoh N, Ao Y, Spence R, Sofroniew MV, et al. Astrocyte CCL2 sustains immune cell infiltration in chronic experimental autoimmune encephalomyelitis. Journal of Neuroimmunology 2014;**274**:53–61

[54] Paul D, Ge S, Lemire Y, Jellison ER, Serwanski DR, Ruddle NH, et al. Cell-selective knockout and 3D confocal image analysis reveals separate roles for astrocyte-and endothelial-derived CCL2 in neuroinflammation. Journal of Neuroinflammation. 2014;**11**

[55] Patani R, Hardingham GE, Liddelow SA. Functional roles of reactive astrocytes in neuroinflammation and

neurodegeneration. Nature Reviews Neurology. 2023;**19**:395–409

[56] He L, Zhang R, Yang M, Lu M. The role of astrocyte in neuroinflammation in traumatic brain injury. Biochimica Et Biophysica Acta (BBA) - Molecular Basis of Disease. 2024;**1870**(4):166992. https://www.sciencedirect.com/science/article/pii/S0925443923003587

[57] McKeon RJ, Jurynec MJ, Buck CR. The chondroitin sulfate proteoglycans neurocan and phosphacan are expressed by reactive astrocytes in the chronic CNS glial scar. Journal of Neuroscience. 1999;**19**(24):10778–10788

[58] Adams KL, Gallo V. The diversity and disparity of the glial scar. Nature Neuroscience. 2018;**21**:9–15

[59] Morgenstern DA, Asher RA, Fawcett JW. Chapter 22 Chondroitin sulphate proteoglycans in the CNS injury response. Progress in Brain Research. 2002;**137**:313–332. https://www.sciencedirect.com/science/article/pii/S0079612302370249?via%3Dihub

[60] Stephenson EL, Yong VW. Pro-inflammatory roles of chondroitin sulfate proteoglycans in disorders of the central nervous system. Matrix Biology: Journal of the International Society for Matrix Biology. 2018;**71–72**:432–442

[61] Yang T, Dai Y, Chen G, Cui S. Dissecting the Dual Role of the Glial Scar and Scar-Forming Astrocytes in Spinal Cord Injury. Frontiers in Cellular Neuroscience. 2020;**14**:78

[62] Lau CL, Kovacevic M, Tingleff TS, Forsythe JS, Cate HS, Merlo D, et al. 3D Electrospun scaffolds promote a cytotrophic phenotype of cultured primary astrocytes. Journal of Neurochemistry 2014;**130**:215–226

[63] Abeysinghe HCS, Phillips EL, Chin-Cheng H, Beart PM, Roulston CL. Modulating astrocyte transition after stroke to promote brain rescue and functional recovery: Emerging targets include Rho Kinase. International Journal of Molecular Sciences. 2016;**17**:288

[64] Cieri MB, Ramos AJ.Astrocytes, reactive astrogliosis, and glial scar formation in traumatic brain injury. Neural Regeneration Research. 2025;**20**(4):973–989

[65] Pekny M, Wilhelmsson U, Pekna M. The dual role of astrocyte activation and reactive gliosis. Neuroscience Letters. 2014;**565**:30–38

[66] Frik J, Merl-Pham J, Plesnila N, Mattugini N, Kjell J, Kraska J, et al. Cross-talk between monocyte invasion and astrocyte proliferation regulates scarring in brain injury. EMBO Reports. 2018;**19**(5):e45294

[67] Dzyubenko E, Manrique-Castano D, Kleinschnitz C, Faissner A, Hermann DM. Role of immune responses for extracellular matrix remodeling in the ischemic brain. Therapeutic Advances in Neurological Disorders. 2018;**11**:1756286418818092

[68] Jones LL, Margolis RU, Tuszynski MH.The chondroitin sulfate proteoglycans neurocan, brevican, phosphacan, and versican are differentially regulated following spinal cord injury. Experimental Neurology. 2003;**182**(2):399–411

[69] Araki T, Ikegaya Y, Koyama R. The effects of microglia- and astrocyte-derived factors on neurogenesis in health and disease. European Journal of Neuroscience. 2021;**54**:5880–5901

[70] Linnerbauer M, Rothhammer V. Protective Functions of Reactive Astrocytes Following Central Nervous System Insult. Frontiers in Immunology. 2020;**11**:573256

[71] Shen XY, Gao ZK, Han Y, Yuan M, Guo YS, Bi X. Activation and Role of Astrocytes in Ischemic Stroke. Frontiers in Cellular Neuroscience. 2021;**15**:755955

[72] Lepore AC, O'donnell J, Kim AS, Yang EJ, Tuteja A, Haidet-Phillips A, et al. Reduction in expression of the astrocyte glutamate transporter, GLT1, worsens functional and histological outcomes following traumatic spinal cord injury. Glia 2011;**59**:1996–2005

[73] Ohno Y, Kunisawa N, Shimizu S. Emerging roles of astrocyte Kir4.1 channels in the pathogenesis and treatment of brain diseases. International Journal of Molecular Sciences. 2021;**22**:10236

[74] Kobayashi E, Nakano M, Kubota K, Himuro N, Mizoguchi S, Chikenji T, et al. Activated forms of astrocytes with higher GLT-1 expression are associated with cognitive normal subjects with Alzheimer pathology in human brain. Scientific Reports. 2018;**8**(1):1712

[75] Liao G, Zhou M, Cheung S, Galeano J, Nguyen N, Baudry M, et al. Reduced early hypoxic/ischemic brain damage is associated with increased GLT-1 levels in mice expressing mutant (P301L) human tau. Brain Research. 2009;**1247**:159–170

[76] Hu B, Pei J, Wan C, Liu S, Xu Z, Zou Y, et al. Mechanisms of postischemic stroke angiogenesis: A multifaceted approach. Journal of Inflammation Research. 2024;**17**:4625–4646

[77] Puebla M, Tapia PJ, Espinoza H. Key role of astrocytes in postnatal brain and retinal angiogenesis. International Journal of Molecular Sciences. 2022;**23**:2646

[78] Miyamoto N, Pham LDD, Seo JH, Kim KW, Lo EH, Arai K. Crosstalk between cerebral endothelium and oligodendrocyte. Cellular and Molecular Life Sciences. 2014;**71**:1055–1066

[79] Bernocchi F, Bonomi CG, Assogna M, Moreschini A, Mercuri NB, Koch G, et al. Astrocytic-derived vascular remodeling factors are independently associated with blood brain barrier permeability in Alzheimer's disease. Neurobiology of Aging. 2024;**141**:66–73. https://www.sciencedirect.com/science/article/pii/S0197458024000940?via%3Dihub

[80] Liu X, Ying J, Wang X, Zheng Q, Zhao T, Yoon S, et al. Astrocytes in neural circuits: Key factors in synaptic regulation and potential targets for neurodevelopmental disorders. Frontiers in Molecular Neuroscience. 2021;**14**:729273

[81] Götz M, Sirko S, Beckers J, Irmler M. Reactive astrocytes as neural stem or progenitor cells: In vivo lineage, In vitro potential, and Genome-wide expression analysis. GLIA. 2015;**63**:1452–1468

[82] Scheib J, Byrd-Jacobs C. Zebrafish astroglial Morphology in the Olfactory bulb is altered with repetitive Peripheral damage. Frontiers in Neuroanatomy. 2020;**14**:14

[83] Goldshmit Y, Sztal TE, Jusuf PR, Hall TE, Nguyen-Chi M, Currie PD.Fgf-dependent glial cell bridges facilitate spinal cord regeneration in Zebrafish. Journal of Neuroscience. 2012;**32**(22):7477–7492

[84] Amlerova Z, Chmelova M, Anderova M, Vargova L. Reactive gliosis in traumatic brain injury: A comprehensive review. Frontiers in Cellular Neuroscience. 2024;**18**:1335849

[85] Li T, Chen X, Zhang C, Zhang Y, Yao W. An update on reactive astrocytes in chronic pain. Journal of Neuroinflammation. 2019;**16**:140

[86] Magnusson JP, Göritz C, Tatarishvili J, Dias DO, Smith EMK, Lindvall O, et al. A latent neurogenic program in astrocytes regulated by Notch signaling in the mouse. Science 2014;**346**:237–241

[87] Kim M, Oh S, Kim S, Kim IS, Kim J, Han J, et al. In vivo neural regeneration via AAV-NeuroD1 gene delivery to astrocytes in neonatal hypoxic-ischemic brain injury. Inflammation and Regeneration 2024;**44**:33

[88] Chen YC, Ma NX, Pei ZF, Wu Z, Do-Monte FH, Keefe S, et al. A NeuroD1 AAV-based gene therapy for functional brain repair after ischemic injury through in vivo Astrocyte-to-neuron conversion. Molecular Therapy 2020;**28**:217–234

[89] Wang Y, Xia Y, Kou L, Yin S, Chi X, Li J, et al. Astrocyte-to-neuron reprogramming and crosstalk in the treatment of Parkinson's disease. Neurobiology of Disease. 2023;**184**:106224

[90] Lang BT, Cregg JM, Depaul MA, Tran AP, Xu K, Dyck SM, et al. Modulation of the proteoglycan receptor PTP σ promotes recovery after spinal cord injury. Nature 2015;**518**:404–408

[91] Francos-Quijorna I, Sánchez-Petidier M, Burnside ER, Badea SR, Torres-Espin A, Marshall L, et al. Chondroitin sulfate proteoglycans prevent immune cell phenotypic conversion and inflammation resolution via TLR4 in rodent models of spinal cord injury. Nature Communications. 2022;**13**(1):2933

[92] Bracchi-Ricard V, Lambertsen KL, Ricard J, Nathanson L, Karmally S, Johnstone J, et al. Inhibition of astroglial NF-kappaB enhances oligodendrogenesis following spinal cord injury. Journal of Neuroinflammation. 2013;**10**:10

[93] Santopolo G, Magnusson JP, Lindvall O, Kokaia Z, Frisén J.Blocking Notch-signaling increases neurogenesis in the striatum after stroke. Cells. 2020;**9**(7):1732

[94] Brambilla R, Hurtado A, Persaud T, Esham K, Pearse DD, Oudega M, et al. Transgenic inhibition of astroglial NF-κB leads to increased axonal sparing and sprouting following spinal cord injury. Journal of Neurochemistry 2009;**110**:765–778

[95] Burda JE, Sofroniew MV. Reactive gliosis and the multicellular response to CNS damage and disease. Neuron. 2014;**81**:229–248

[96] Sun M, You H, Hu X, Luo Y, Zhang Z, Song Y, et al. Microglia–astrocyte interaction in neural development and neural pathogenesis. Cells. 2023;**12**:1942

[97] Norden DM, Trojanowski PJ, Villanueva E, Navarro E, Godbout JP. Sequential activation of microglia and astrocyte cytokine expression precedes increased iba-1 or GFAP immunoreactivity following systemic immune challenge. Glia. 2016;**64**(2):300–316

[98] Renault-Mihara F, Mukaino M, Shinozaki M, Kumamaru H, Kawase S, Baudoux M, et al. Regulation of RhoA by STAT3 coordinates glial scar formation. Journal of Cell Biology 2017;**216**:2533–2550

[99] Norden DM, Fenn AM, Dugan A, Godbout JP.TGFβ produced by IL-10 redirected astrocytes attenuates microglial activation. Glia. 2014;**62** (6):881–895

[100] Jung BK, Ryu KY. Lipocalin-2: A therapeutic target to overcome neurodegenerative diseases by regulating reactive astrogliosis. Experimental and Molecular Medicine. 2023;**55**:2138–2146

[101] Tan Q, Zhang C, Rao X, Wan W, Lin W, Huang S, et al. The interaction of lipocalin-2 and astrocytes in neuroinflammation: Mechanisms and therapeutic application. Frontiers in Immunology. 2024;**15**:1358719

[102] Pawelec P, Ziemka-Nalecz M, Sypecka J, Zalewska T. The impact of the cx3cl1/cx3cr1 axis in neurological disorders. Cells. 2020;**9**:2277

[103] Shrivastava K, Gonzalez P, Acarin L.The immune inhibitory complex CD200/CD200R is developmentally regulated in the mouse brain. Journal of Comparative Neurology. 2012;**520** (12):2657–2675

[104] Schröder LJ, Mulenge F, Pavlou A, Skripuletz T, Stangel M, Gudi V, et al. Dynamics of reactive astrocytes fosters tissue regeneration after cuprizone-induced demyelination. Glia 2023;**71**:2573–2590

[105] Catalano M, Lauro C, Cipriani R, Chece G, Ponzetta A, Di Angelantonio S, et al. CX3CL1 protects neurons against excitotoxicity enhancing GLT-1 activity on astrocytes. Journal of Neuroimmunology 2013;**263**:75–82

[106] Koizumi S, Fujishita K, Inoue K. Regulation of cell-to-cell communication mediated by astrocytic ATP in the CNS. Purinergic Signalling. 2005;**1**:211–217

[107] Agulhon C, Sun MY, Murphy T, Myers T, Lauderdale K, Fiacco TA. Calcium signaling and gliotransmission in normal vs. Reactive astrocytes. Frontiers in Pharmacology. 2012;**3**:139

[108] Pöyhönen S, Er S, Domanskyi A, Airavaara M. Effects of neurotrophic factors in glial cells in the central nervous system: Expression and properties in neurodegeneration and injury. Frontiers in Physiology. 2019;**10**:486

[109] Toyomoto M, Inoue S, Ohta K, Kuno S, Ohta M, Hayashi K, et al. Production of NGF, BDNF and GDNF in mouse astrocyte cultures is strongly enhanced by a cerebral vasodilator, ifenprodil. Neuroscience Letters. 2005;**379**(3):185–189

[110] Pajarillo E, Rizor A, Lee J, Aschner M, Lee E. The role of astrocytic glutamate transporters GLT-1 and GLAST in neurological disorders: Potential targets for neurotherapeutics. Neuropharmacology. 2019;**161**:107559

[111] Yi JH, Hazell AS.Excitotoxic mechanisms and the role of astrocytic glutamate transporters in traumatic brain injury. Neurochemistry International. 2006;**48**(5):394–403

[112] O'Donovan SM, Sullivan CR, McCullumsmith RE. The role of

glutamate transporters in the pathophysiology of neuropsychiatric disorders. Npj Schizophrenia. 2017;**3**:32

[113] Halassa MM, Fellin T, Haydon PG. The tripartite synapse: Roles for gliotransmission in health and disease. Trends in Molecular Medicine. 2007;**13** (2):54–63

[114] Perea G, Navarrete M, Araque A. Tripartite synapses: Astrocytes process and control synaptic information. Trends in Neurosciences. 2009;**32**:421–431

[115] Kang N, Peng H, Yu Y, Stanton PK, Guilarte TR, Kang J. Astrocytes release d-serine by a large vesicle. Neuroscience. 2013;**240**:243–257

[116] Goenaga J, Araque A, Kofuji P, Herrera Moro Chao D. Calcium signaling in astrocytes and gliotransmitter release. Frontiers in Synaptic Neuroscience. 2023;**15**:1138577

[117] Bai Y, Zhou Z, Han B, Xiang X, Huang W, Yao H. Revisiting astrocytic calcium signaling in the brain. Fundamental Research. 2024;**4**:1365–1374

[118] Pellerin L, Pellegri G, Bittar PG, Charnay Y, Bouras C, Martin JL, et al. Evidence supporting the existence of an activity-dependent astrocyte-neuron lactate shuttle. Developmental Neuroscience. 1998;**20**:291–299

[119] Pellerin L, Bouzier-Sore AK, Aubert A, Serres S, Merle M, Costalat R, et al. Activity-dependent regulation of energy metabolism by astrocytes: An update. GLIA. 2007;**55**:1251–1262

[120] Suzuki A, Stern SA, Bozdagi O, Huntley GW, Walker RH, Magistretti PJ, et al. Astrocyte-neuron lactate transport is required for long-term memory formation. Cell 2011;**144**:810–823

[121] Olsen ML, Sontheimer H. Functional implications for Kir4.1 channels in glial biology: From K + buffering to cell differentiation. Journal of Neurochemistry. 2008;**107**:589–601

[122] Kinboshi M, Ikeda A, Ohno Y. Role of Astrocytic Inwardly Rectifying Potassium (Kir) 4.1 Channels in Epileptogenesis. Frontiers in Neurology. 2020;**11**:626658

[123] Rawji KS, Gonzalez Martinez GA, Sharma A, Franklin RJM. The Role of Astrocytes in Remyelination. Trends in Neurosciences. 2020;**43**;(8):596–607

[124] Ishibashi T, Lee PR, Baba H, Fields RD.Leukemia inhibitory factor regulates the timing of oligodendrocyte development and myelination in the postnatal optic nerve. Journal of Neuroscience Research. 2009;**87** (15):3343–3355

[125] Harlow DE, Macklin WB. Inhibitors of myelination: ECM changes, CSPGs and PTPs. Experimental Neurology. 2014;**251**:39–46

[126] Lau LW, Keough MB, Haylock-Jacobs S, Cua R, Döring A, Sloka S, et al. Chondroitin sulfate proteoglycans in demyelinated lesions impair remyelination. Annals of Neurology. 2012;**72**(3):23599

[127] Aharoni R, Eilam R, Arnon R. Astrocytes in multiple sclerosis—essential constituents with diverse multifaceted functions. International Journal of Molecular Sciences. 2021;**22**:5904

[128] Molina-Gonzalez I, Holloway RK, Jiwaji Z, Dando O, Kent SA, Emelianova K, et al. Astrocyte-oligodendrocyte interaction regulates central nervous system regeneration. Nature Communications. 2023;**14**(1):3372

[129] Domingues HS, Portugal CC, Socodato R, Relvas JB. Oligodendrocyte, astrocyte, and microglia crosstalk in myelin development, damage, and repair. Frontiers in Cell and Developmental Biology. 2016;**4**:71

[130] Ghézali G, Ribot J, Curry N, Pillet L, Boutet-Porretta F, Mozheiko D, et al. Connexin 30 locally controls actin cytoskeleton and mechanical remodeling in motile astrocytes. Glia 2024;**72**:1915–1929

[131] Le HT, Sin WC, Lozinsky S, Bechberger J, Vega JL, Guo XQ, et al. Gap junction intercellular communication mediated by connexin43 in astrocytes is essential for their resistance to oxidative stress. Journal of Biological Chemistry. 2014;**289**(3):1345–1354

[132] Xu H, Li H, Zhang P, Gao Y, Ma H, Gao T, et al. The functions of exosomes targeting astrocytes and astrocyte-derived exosomes targeting other cell types. Neural Regeneration Research. 2024;**19**:1947–53

[133] Ogaki A, Ikegaya Y, Koyama R. Extracellular vesicles taken up by astrocytes. International Journal of Molecular Sciences. 2021;**22**:10553

[134] Li F, Kang X, Xin W, Li X. The Emerging Role of Extracellular Vesicle Derived From Neurons/Neurogliocytes in Central Nervous System Diseases: Novel Insights Into Ischemic Stroke. Frontiers in Pharmacology. 2022;**13**:890698

[135] Chen C, Shu Y, Yan C, Li H, Huang Z, Shen S, et al. Astrocyte-derived clusterin disrupts glial physiology to obstruct remyelination in mouse models of demyelinating diseases. Nature Communications 2024;**15**:7791

[136] Liu CY, Yang Y, Ju WN, Wang X, Zhang HL. Emerging roles of astrocytes in neuro-vascular unit and the tripartite synapse with emphasis on reactive gliosis in the context of Alzheimer's disease. Frontiers in Cellular Neuroscience. 2018;**12**:193

[137] Han G, Song L, Ding Z, Wang Q, Yan Y, Huang J, et al. The Important Double-Edged Role of Astrocytes in Neurovascular Unit After Ischemic Stroke. Frontiers in Aging Neuroscience. 2022;**14**:833431

[138] Gong Y, Wu M, Huang Y, He X, Yuan J, Dang B.Research developments in the neurovascular unit and the blood-brain barrier (Review). Biomed Reports. 2025;**22**(5):1–14

[139] Liu LR, Liu JC, Bao JS, Bai QQ, Wang GQ. Interaction of Microglia and Astrocytes in the Neurovascular Unit. Frontiers in Immunology. 2020;**11**:1024

[140] Schiera G, Di Liegro CM, Schirò G, Sorbello G, Di Liegro I. Involvement of Astrocytes in the Formation, Maintenance, and Function of the Blood–Brain Barrier. Cells. 2024;**13**:150

[141] Michinaga S, Koyama Y. Dual roles of astrocyte-derived factors in regulation of blood-brain barrier function after brain damage. International Journal of Molecular Sciences. 2019;**20**:571

[142] Egervari K, Potter G, Guzman-Hernandez ML, Salmon P, Soto-Ribeiro

M, Kastberger B, et al. Astrocytes spatially restrict VEGF signaling by polarized secretion and incorporation of VEGF into the actively assembling extracellular matrix. Glia 2016;**64**:440–456

[143] Cheng J, Zheng Y, Cheng F, Wang C, Han J, Zhang H, et al. Different roles of astrocytes in the blood-brain barrier during the acute and recovery phases of stroke. Neural Regeneration Research. 2025;**21**:1359–1372

[144] Feng XF, Li MC, ZY L, Li MZ, Lu Y, Zhuang YM, et al. Tetramethylpyrazine promotes stroke recovery by inducing the restoration of neurovascular unit and transformation of A1/A2 reactive astrocytes. Frontiers in Cellular Neuroscience. 2023;170:105607

[145] Swissa E, Serlin Y, Vazana U, Prager O, Friedman A. Blood–brain barrier dysfunction in status epileptics: Mechanisms and role in epileptogenesis. Epilepsy and Behavior. 2019;**101**:106285

[146] Berezowski V, Fukuda AM, Cecchelli R, Badaut J. Endothelial Cells and Astrocytes: A Concerto en Duo in Ischemic Pathophysiology. International Journal of Cell Biology. 2012;**2012**:1–16

[147] Che J, Sun Y, Deng Y, Zhang J. Blood-brain barrier disruption: A culprit of cognitive decline? Fluids and Barriers of the CNS. 2024;**21**(1):63

[148] Manu DR, Slevin M, Barcutean L, Forro T, Boghitoiu T, Balasa R. Astrocyte Involvement in Blood–Brain Barrier Function: A Critical Update Highlighting Novel, Complex, Neurovascular Interactions. International Journal of Molecular Sciences. 2023;**24**:17146

[149] Pringle AK, Solomon E, Coles BJ, Desousa BR, Shtaya A, Gajavelli S, et al. Sonic Hedgehog Signaling Promotes Peri-Lesion Cell Proliferation and Functional Improvement after Cortical Contusion Injury. Neurotrauma Reports 2021;**2**:27–38

[150] Tail M, Zhang H, Zheng G, Hatami M, Skutella T, Unterberg A, et al. The Sonic Hedgehog Pathway Modulates Survival, Proliferation, and Differentiation of Neural Progenitor Cells under Inflammatory Stress In Vitro. 2022;**11**(4):736

[151] Arredondo SB, Valenzuela-Bezanilla D, Mardones MD, Varela-Nallar L. Role of Wnt Signaling in Adult Hippocampal Neurogenesis in Health and Disease. Frontiers in Cell and Developmental Biology. 2020;**8**:860

[152] Varela-Nallar L, Inestrosa NC. Wnt signaling in the regulation of adult hippocampal neurogenesis. Frontiers in Cellular Neuroscience. 2013;**7** (JUNE):100

[153] Lampada A, Taylor V. Notch signaling as a master regulator of adult neurogenesis. Frontiers in Neuroscience. 2023;**17**:1179011

[154] Stackhouse TL, Mishra A. Neurovascular Coupling in Development and Disease: Focus on Astrocytes. Frontiers in Cell and Developmental Biology. 2021;**9**:702832

[155] Hösli L, Zuend M, Bredell G, Zanker HS, Porto de Oliveira CE, Saab AS, et al. Direct vascular contact is a hallmark of cerebral astrocytes. Cell Reports 2022;**39**:110599

[156] Long KR, Huttner WB. How the extracellular matrix shapes neural

development. Open Biology. 2019;**9**:180216

[157] Woo AM, Sontheimer H. Interactions between astrocytes and extracellular matrix structures contribute to neuroinflammation-associated epilepsy pathology. Frontiers in Molecular Medicine. 2023;3:1198021

[158] Gong S, Shao H, Cai X, Zhu J. Astrocyte-Derived Neuronal Transdifferentiation as a Therapy for Ischemic Stroke: Advances and Challenges. Brain Sciences. 2022;**12**:1175

[159] Yang H, Cheng XP, Li JW, Yao Q, Ju G.De-differentiation response of cultured astrocytes to injury induced by scratch or conditioned culture medium of scratch-insulted astrocytes. Cellular and Molecular Neurobiology. 2009;**29** (4):455–473

[160] Huang M, Long A, Hao L, Shi Z, Zhang M. Astrocyte in Neurological Disease: Pathogenesis and Therapy. MedComm (Beijing). 2025;**6**(8): e70299

[161] Todd AC, Hardingham GE. The regulation of astrocytic glutamate transporters in health and neurodegenerative diseases. International Journal of Molecular Sciences. 2020;**21**:9607

[162] Muñoz de León-lópez CA, Navarro-Lobato I, Khan ZU.The Role of Astrocytes in Synaptic Dysfunction and Memory Deficits in Alzheimer's Disease. Biomolecules. 2025;**15**(7):910

[163] Chung WS, Clarke LE, Wang GX, Stafford BK, Sher A, Chakraborty C, et al. Astrocytes mediate synapse elimination through MEGF10 and MERTK pathways. Nature 2013;**504**:394–400

[164] Dejanovic B, Wu T, Tsai MC, Graykowski D, Gandham VD, Rose CM, et al. Complement C1q-dependent excitatory and inhibitory synapse elimination by astrocytes and microglia in Alzheimer's disease mouse models. Nature Aging 2022;**2**:837–850

[165] Brucato FH, Benjamin DE. Synaptic Pruning in Alzheimer's Disease: Role of the Complement System. Global Journal of Medical Research. 2020;**20**:1–20

[166] Ding X, Wang J, Huang M, Chen Z, Liu J, Zhang Q, et al. Loss of microglial SIRPα promotes synaptic pruning in preclinical models of neurodegeneration. Nature Communications. 2021;**12**(1):2030

[167] Liu H, Jiang M, Chen Z, Li C, Yin X, Zhang X, et al. The Role of the Complement System in Synaptic Pruning after Stroke. Aging and Disease. 2024;**16**(3):1452–1470

[168] Cassé F, Richetin K, Toni N. Astrocytes' contribution to adult neurogenesis in physiology and Alzheimer's disease. Frontiers in Cellular Neuroscience. 2018;**12**:432

[169] Jiao J, Chen DF.Induction of Neurogenesis in Nonconventional Neurogenic Regions of the Adult Central Nervous System by Niche Astrocyte-Produced Signals. Stem Cells. 2008;**26**(5):1221–1230

[170] Gengatharan A, Bammann RR, Saghatelyan A. The role of astrocytes in the generation, migration, and integration of new neurons in the adult olfactory bulb. Frontiers in Neuroscience. 2016;**10**:149

[171] Bielefeld P, Martirosyan A, Martín-Suárez S, Apresyan A, Meerhoff

GF, Pestana F, et al. Traumatic brain injury promotes neurogenesis at the cost of astrogliogenesis in the adult hippocampus of male mice. Nature Communications 2024;**15**:5222

[172] Wu X, Chen PS, Dallas S, Wilson B, Block ML, Wang CC, et al. Histone deacetylase inhibitors up-regulate astrocyte GDNF and BDNF gene transcription and protect dopaminergic neurons. International Journal of Neuropsychopharmacology 2008;**11**:1123

[173] Talifu Z, Liu JY, Pan YZ, Ke H, Zhang CJ, Xu X, et al. In vivo astrocyte-to-neuron reprogramming for central nervous system regeneration: A narrative review. Neural Regeneration Research. 2023;**18**:750–755

[174] Ohtake Y, Li S. Molecular mechanisms of scar-sourced axon growth inhibitors. Brain Research. 2015;**1619**:22–35

[175] Hosseini SM, Alizadeh A, Shahsavani N, Chopek J, Ahlfors JE, Karimi-Abdolrezaee S.Suppressing CSPG/LAR/PTP σ Axis Facilitates Neuronal Replacement and Synaptogenesis by Human Neural Precursor Grafts and Improves Recovery after Spinal Cord Injury. The Journal of Neuroscience. 2022;**42** (15):3096–3121

[176] Ikegami T, Nakamura M, Yamane J, Katoh H, Okada S, Iwanami A, et al. Chondroitinase ABC combined with neural stem/progenitor cell transplantation enhances graft cell migration and outgrowth of growth-associated protein-43-positive fibers after rat spinal cord injury. European Journal of Neuroscience 2005;**22**:3036–3046

[177] Bormann D, Knoflach M, Poreba E, Riedl CJ, Testa G, Orset C, et al. Single-nucleus RNA sequencing reveals glial cell type-specific responses to ischemic stroke in male rodents. Nature Communications 2024;**15**:6232

[178] Santos DE, Silva Lima SA, Moreira LS, Lima Costa S, de Sampaio Schitine C. New perspectives on heterogeneity in astrocyte reactivity in neuroinflammation. Brain, Behavior, and Immunity - Health. 2025;**44**:100948. Available from: https://www.sciencedirect.com/science/article/pii/S2666354625000067?via%3Dihub [Accessed: 2025-July-07]

[179] Wanner IB, Anderson MA, Song B, Levine J, Fernandez A, Gray-Thompson Z, et al. Glial Scar Borders Are Formed by Newly Proliferated, Elongated Astrocytes That Interact to Corral Inflammatory and Fibrotic Cells via STAT3-Dependent Mechanisms after Spinal Cord Injury. Journal of Neuroscience 2013;**33**:12870–12886

[180] Chalmers N, Masouti E, Beckervordersandforth R. Astrocytes in the adult dentate gyrus—balance between adult and developmental tasks. Molecular Psychiatry. 2024;**29**:982–991

[181] Yang H, An J, Choi I, Lee K, Park SM, Jou I, et al. Region-specific astrogliosis: Differential vessel formation contributes to different patterns of astrogliosis in the cortex and striatum. Molecular Brain. 2020;**13** (1):103

[182] Ding S. Dynamic reactive astrocytes after focal ischemia. Neural Regeneration Research. 2014;**9**:2048

[183] Anderson MA, Burda JE, Ren Y, Ao Y, O'Shea TM, Kawaguchi R, et al. Astrocyte scar formation AIDS central nervous system axon regeneration. Nature 2016;**532**:195–200

[184] Lee HG, Rone JM, Li Z, Akl CF, Shin SW, Lee JH, et al. Disease-associated astrocyte epigenetic memory promotes CNS pathology. Nature. 2024;**627**(8005):865–872

[185] Williamson MR, Deneen B. Astrocytes remember inflammation. Immunity. 2024;**57**(5):938–940. https://www.sciencedirect.com/science/article/pii/S1074761324002103

[186] Hennessy E, Griffin EW, Cunningham C.Astrocytes are primed by chronic neurodegeneration to produce exaggerated chemokine and cell infiltration responses to acute stimulation with the cytokines IL-1β and TNF-α. Journal of Neuroscience. 2015;**35**(22):8411–8422

[187] Bradbury EJ, Burnside ER. Moving beyond the glial scar for spinal cord repair. Nature Communications. 2019;**10**:3879

[188] Gu Y, Cheng X, Huang X, Yuan Y, Qin S, Tan Z, et al. Conditional ablation of reactive astrocytes to dissect their roles in spinal cord injury and repair. Brain, Behavior, and Immunity. 2019;**80**:394–405. https://www.sciencedirect.com/science/article/pii/S0889159118303118?utm_source=chatgpt.com

[189] Costa G, Ribeiro FF, Sebastião AM, Muir EM, Vaz SH. Bridging the gap of axonal regeneration in the central nervous system: A state of the art review on central axonal regeneration. Frontiers in Neuroscience. 2022;**16**:1003145

[190] Ben HL, Ceyzériat K, de Sauvage MAC, Aubry F, Auregan G, Guillermier M, et al. The JAK/STAT3 pathway is a common inducer of astrocyte reactivity in Alzheimer's and Huntington's diseases. Journal of Neuroscience. 2015;**35**(6):2817–2829

[191] Liu B, Chen H, Johns TG, Neufeld AH.Epidermal growth factor receptor activation: An upstream signal for transition of quiescent astrocytes into reactive astrocytes after neural injury. Journal of Neuroscience. 2006;**26** (28):7532–7540

[192] Guo R, Han D, Song X, Gao Y, Li Z, Li X, et al. Context-dependent regulation of Notch signaling in glial development and tumorigenesis. Science Advances. 2023;**9**(45):eadi2167

[193] Li CY, Li X, Liu SF, Qu WS, Wang W, Tian DS. Inhibition of mTOR pathway restrains astrocyte proliferation, migration and production of inflammatory mediators after oxygen-glucose deprivation and reoxygenation. Neurochemistry International. 2015;**89**:83–84

[194] Guo Z, Zhang L, Wu Z, Chen Y, Wang F, Chen G.In vivo direct reprogramming of reactive glial cells into functional neurons after brain injury and in an alzheimer's disease model. Cell Stem Cell. 2014;**14**(2):188–202

[195] Niu W, Zang T, Smith DK, Vue TY, Zou Y, Bachoo R, et al. SOX2 reprograms resident astrocytes into neural progenitors in the adult brain. Stem Cell Reports 2015;**4**:780–794

[196] Zhang L, Yin JC, Yeh H, Ma NX, Lee G, Chen XA, et al. Small Molecules Efficiently Reprogram Human Astroglial Cells into Functional Neurons. Cell Stem Cell 2015;**17**:735–747

[197] Bajohr J, Scott EY, Olfat A, Sadria M, Lee K, Fahim M, et al. Direct lineage conversion of postnatal mouse cortical

astrocytes to oligodendrocyte lineage cells. 2024

[198] Khanghahi AM, Satarian L, Deng W, Baharvand H, Javan M. In vivo conversion of astrocytes into oligodendrocyte lineage cells with transcription factor Sox10; Promise for myelin repair in multiple sclerosis. PLoS One. 2018;**13**(9):e0203785

[199] Sharifi-Kelishadi M, Zare L, Fathollahi Y, Javan M.Conversion of astrocyte cell lines to oligodendrocyte progenitor cells using small molecules and transplantation to animal model of Multiple Sclerosis. Journal of Molecular Neuroscience. 2024;**74**(2):40

[200] Nakano-Kobayashi A, Canela A, Yoshihara T, Hagiwara M. Astrocyte-targeting therapy rescues cognitive impairment caused by neuroinflammation via the Nrf2 pathway. Proceedings of the National Academy of Sciences of the United States of America. 2023;**120**(33): e2303809120

[201] Gradišnik L, Bošnjak R, Maver T, Velnar T. Advanced bio-based polymers for astrocyte cell models. Materials. 2021;**14**:3664

[202] Mofrad YM, Asiaei S, Shaygani H, Cheraghi F, Amirsadat S, Soltani M, et al. Advances in smart hydrogels for Nerve repair: A review focusing on criteria and applications. Journal of Science: Advanced Materials and Devices. 2025;**100996**. https://linkinghub.elsevier.com/retrieve/pii/S2468217925001492

[203] Liddelow SA, Barres BA. Reactive Astrocytes: Production, Function, and Therapeutic Potential. Immunity. 2017;**46**:957–967

[204] Matusova Z, Hol EM, Pekny M, Kubista M, Valihrach L. Reactive astrogliosis in the era of single-cell transcriptomics. Frontiers in Cellular Neuroscience. 2023;**17**:1173200

Section 5

Glial Cell Neurodegeneration

Chapter 5

How Glial Cell Dysfunction Fuels Neurodegeneration in Alzheimer's and Prion Diseases? Emerging Targets for Therapy

Saima Zafar, Urwah Rasheed and Inga Zerr

Abstract

Neurodegenerative diseases, including Alzheimer's disease (AD) and prion disorders, have historically been studied from a neuron-centric perspective. However, growing evidence highlights glial cells – particularly microglia and astrocytes – as central mediators of disease initiation and progression. Glia maintain central nervous system homeostasis through waste clearance, synaptic regulation, metabolic support, and blood–brain barrier maintenance. In pathological contexts, glial populations undergo morphological and functional changes, commonly termed reactive gliosis, which can be either protective or detrimental depending on the disease stage. In AD, microglial dysfunction impairs amyloid clearance, promotes chronic cytokine release, and contributes to synaptic loss, while reactive astrocytes exacerbate glutamate excitotoxicity and metabolic dysregulation. Similarly, prion diseases demonstrate that glial cells mediate neurotoxicity and pathogen propagation, with astrocytes showing transcriptomic alterations preceding neuronal demise and microglial ablation paradoxically accelerating disease. Shared pathomechanisms between AD and prion diseases include mitochondrial dysfunction, inflammasome activation, cytokine network dysregulation, and impaired phagocytosis, with the NLRP3 inflammasome emerging as a key therapeutic target. Recent advances in single-cell transcriptomics and spatial proteomics are elucidating the molecular heterogeneity of reactive glia, paving the way for precision medicine approaches. Given the challenges of directly targeting misfolded proteins, glia-focused therapies – ranging from anti-inflammatory agents to gene therapy – represent a promising avenue. This chapter reviews the multifaceted roles of glial cells in neurodegeneration, emphasizing how chronic activation, impaired signaling, and genetic susceptibility convert protective functions into drivers of neuronal dysfunction, and explores emerging strategies for glia-targeted interventions in AD and prion diseases.

Keywords: glial cells, Alzheimer's disease, prion diseases, neurodegeneration, neuroinflammation, reactive gliosis, microglia, astrocytes, therapeutic targets, protein misfolding

1. Introduction

Neurodegenerative diseases, including Alzheimer's disease (AD) and prion diseases, are characterized by progressive neuronal loss, synaptic dysfunction, and the accumulation of misfolded proteins [1]. Traditionally, these disorders have been viewed through a neuron-centric lens. However, growing evidence has repositioned glial cells, particularly astrocytes and microglia, as central players in the pathogenesis and progression of neurodegeneration [2]. Far from being passive bystanders, glial cells actively shape disease environments through inflammatory signaling, failed clearance of pathological proteins, and dysfunctional metabolic support [3, 4].

Glial cells are required for the homeostatic maintenance of the central nervous system (CNS) [5]. The resident immune cell in the brain, the microglia, actively monitors the brain environment, clears waste, and regulates synaptic elimination during development and disease [6]. The most common glial subpopulation, astrocytes, mediate the presence of neurotransmitters, ion equilibrium, energy production, and blood–brain barrier (BBB) health [7]. Oligodendrocytes offer support factors and enable the swift transmission of signals through myelination. In pathological situations, such glial populations experience morphological and functional modifications, usually considered together as the process of gliosis or reactive gliosis, which may be beneficial or harmful depending on the nature of a disease and its temporal progression [8].

Neuroinflammation has been established as a central pathological determinant in AD, and glial cells have found themselves in the limelight in terms of disease progression. The presence of several AD risk genes that are mainly expressed in microglia (TREM2, CD33, and CR1) supports the role of innate immune signaling in susceptibility to the disease, as detected in genome-wide association studies (GWASs) [9]. Dysfunction of microglia causes abnormal clearance of amyloid plaques, over-secretion of cytokines, and loss of synapses. Similarly, astrocytes become reactive and are no longer able to maintain homeostatic activity, a factor that promotes glutamate excitotoxicity and dysregulation of metabolism [10]. The current paradigm shift regarding AD research identifies that glial dysfunction is not only a by-product of the disorder but could also be among the initial and driving causes of neurodegeneration.

Protein misfolding and glial involvement can be better viewed through prion diseases, albeit lesser frequency. Under such conditions, a template-like conformational conversion facilitates the spread of misfolded prion protein (PrP 23), causing massive neurotoxicity. It is remarkable that prion replication and neurodegeneration may develop independently of a substantial adaptive immune response, suggesting that both innate immune cells, in particular microglia and astrocytes, are important mediators of the pathogenesis [11]. The ablation of microglia in mouse models of prion disease has similarly been paradoxically shown to accelerate progression, suggesting a dual role of microglia in neurotoxicity as well as neuroprotection [12]. Astrocytes are another type of cell that contain PrPSc; they also have transcriptomic alterations that precede neuronal demise, hinting at them being the main agents of pathogen propagation and toxicity [13].

One commonality between AD and prion illnesses is the presence of glial phenotypes associated with a patho-mechanistic framework, such as mitochondrial dysfunction, cytokine network dysregulation, inflammasome activation, and impaired phagocytosis. An example is provided by the NLRP3 inflammasome, which has proven that its stimulation in microglia provokes chronic inflammation as well as neuronal damage. NLRP3 and its downstream effectors are therapeutically viable in preclinical models of AD and prion disease [14]. Similarly, it has been demonstrated that manipulating microglial receptors like TREM2 is sufficient to reshape glial reactions and reduce the illness burden [15].

Given the difficulties in directly targeting misfolded proteins, therapeutic approaches that target glial cells present a possible path for intervention. These strategies include repurposing anti-inflammatory drugs, gene therapy, small compounds, and monoclonal antibodies. A major obstacle, though, is the variation in glial responses throughout illness stages and brain areas. The intricate molecular markers of reactive glia are being deciphered through recent developments in single-cell transcriptomics and spatial proteomics, opening the door for precision medicine techniques [16].

This chapter focuses on the multifaceted roles of glial cells in AD and prion diseases (**Figure 1**). It outlines how their protective functions are undermined by chronic activation, impaired signaling, and genetic susceptibility. Furthermore, it examines how glia contribute to both the propagation of neurotoxicity and the modulation of synaptic integrity, and how this understanding may lead to novel glia-targeted therapeutic strategies.

2. Astrocytes in Alzheimer's disease

The most common glial cells in the CNS are astrocytes, which play a central role in maintaining the CNS by regulating neurotransmitter clearance, ion buffering, brain–blood flow, and metabolism [7]. The star-shaped cells are also crucial in synapse development, elimination, and support [17]. Astrocytes in AD undergo extensive functional and morphological modifications, known as reactive astrocytosis, which is accompanied by an increase in glial fibrillary acidic protein (GFAP) expression, cellular hypertrophy, proliferation, and the release of inflammatory molecules [18].

Although the initial stimulation of astrocyte cells is defensive in nature (intending to regain CNS balance), continuous stimulation causes the loss of supportive roles and the escalation of inflammation, which promotes the development of diseases [19]. Below, we explore the multifaceted role of astrocytes in AD pathogenesis.

2.1 Interaction with amyloid-β

The key underlying pathology of AD is the production of plaques from amyloid-β (Aβ) aggregation. Astrocytes play a dual and time-dependent role in Aβ metabolism, as depicted in **Figure 2**. In the initial phases, the astrocytes engulf Aβ via the low-density lipoprotein receptor-related protein 1 (LRP1) receptor and degrade it through the lysosomal mechanism, thus reducing the formation of plaques [20, 21]. However, as the disease progresses, the ability of astrocytes to clear Aβ also diminishes. Aβ plaques are surrounded by reactive astrocytes that have taken on a pro-inflammatory appearance and secrete cytokines such as IL-1β, TNF-α, and IL-6 [22]. This inflammatory environment in the nervous tissue increases synaptic dysfunction as well as neuronal damage.

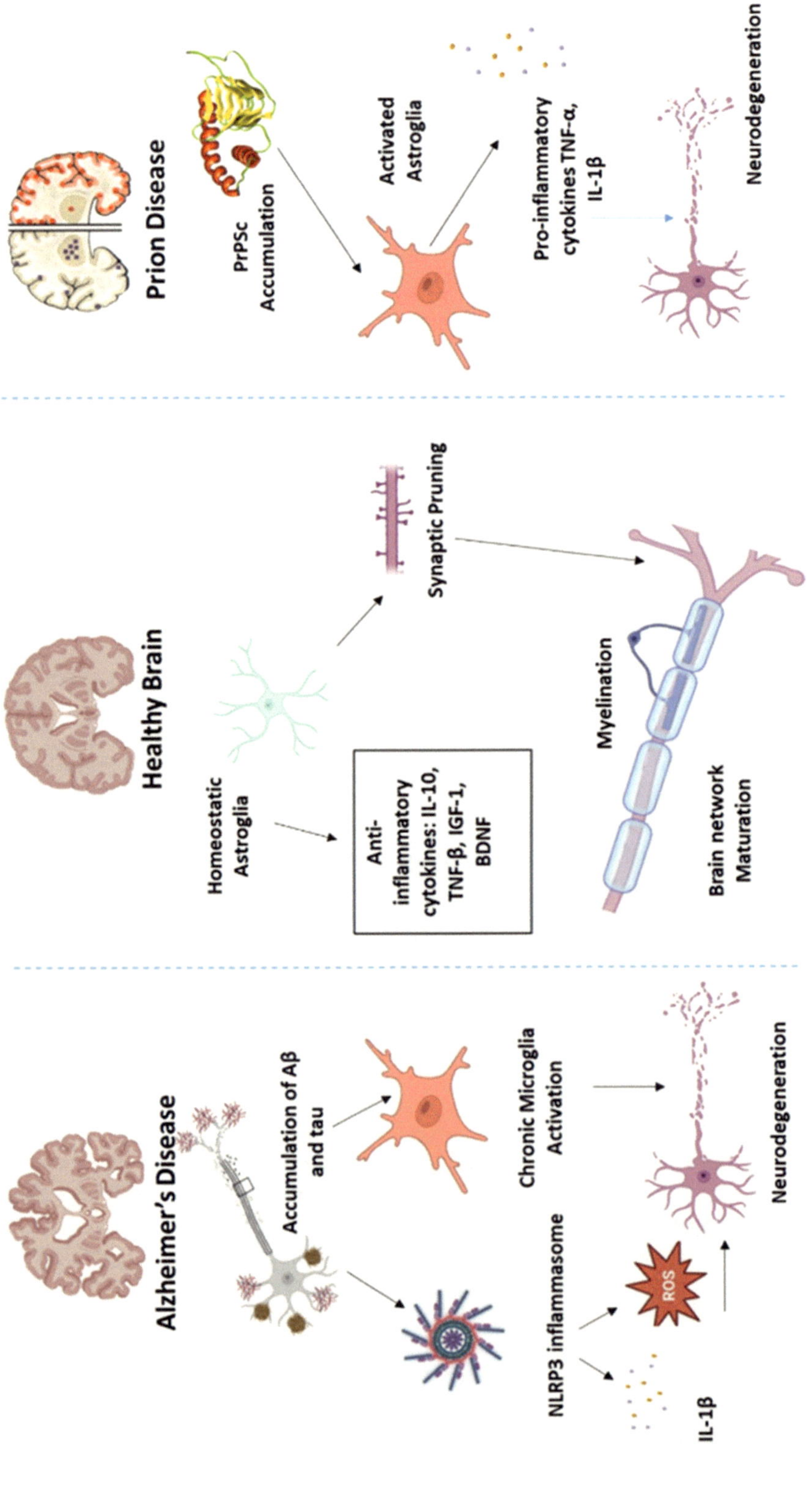

Figure 1.
The figure depicts how glial cells and inflammatory pathways function differently in neurodegeneration in a healthy brain as opposed to an AD-affected brain (driven by Aβ, tau, and the NLRP3 inflammasome) and a prion disease-affected brain (driven by PrPSc and activated astroglia).

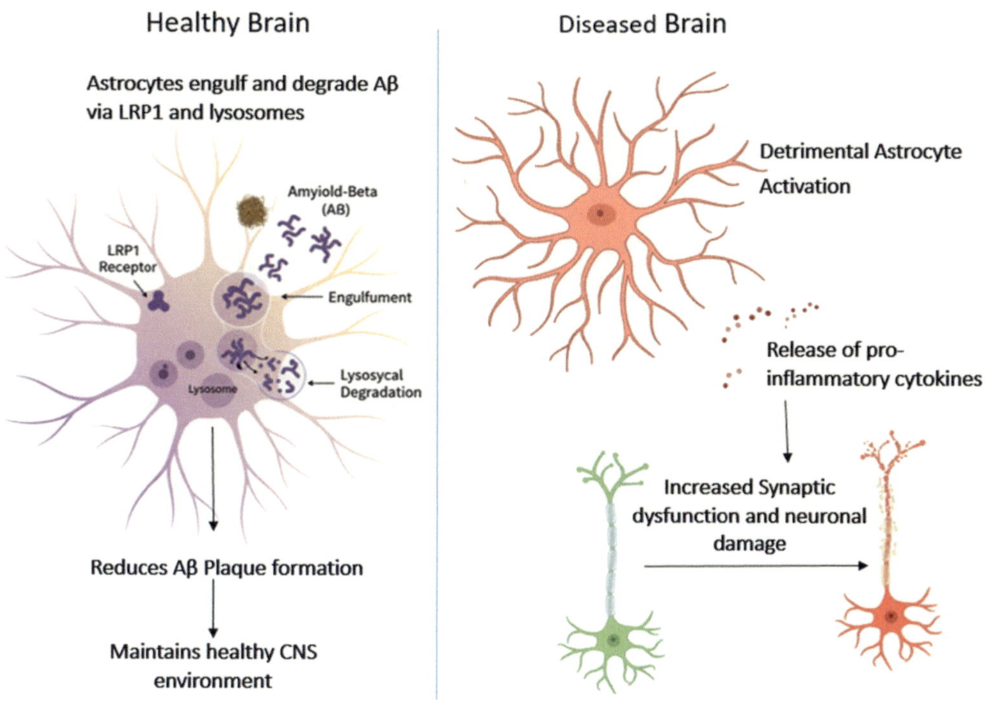

Figure 2.
Astrocyte function in health and diseased brain. Healthy astrocytes clear Aβ to maintain CNS balance, while diseased astrocytes release inflammatory cytokines causing neuronal damage.

Furthermore, astrocytes themselves contain intracellular Aβ, which disrupts the lysosomal activity of the cell and hence worsens the oxidative stress condition [23]. Recently, transcriptomic analyses have been used to describe Aβ-induced astrocytic subpopulations (e.g., disease-associated astrocytes, or DAA), which have dysregulated expression of genes related to CNS inflammation, lipid metabolism, and phagocytosis [24].

2.2 Glutamate dysregulation and excitotoxicity

Astrocytes also play a role in controlling synaptic glutamate homeostasis through the expression of excitatory amino acid transporters, of which EAAT2 (GLT1 in rodents) constitutes more than 90% of brain glutamate uptake [25]. In animal models, impaired EAAT2 clearance and low expression are shown in the brains of humans and animals [26].

This excitotoxicity caused by glutamate leads to calcium overloading, oxidative stress, and finally neuronal apoptosis. Additionally, Aβ oligomers have been shown to impair EAAT2 expression via epigenetic mechanisms and by inducing oxidative modifications on transporter proteins [27]. Hence, therapeutic approaches that may be used to increase the expression or activity of EAAT2 will provide a potential benefit in reducing excitotoxic injury in AD models.

2.3 Astrocytic metabolic failure

Astrocytes normally support neurons through lactate shuttle mechanisms and glycogen metabolism [28]. In AD, astrocytic metabolic function declines, contributing to energy deficits in neurons and reduced resilience to toxic stress [29]. The astrocyte-neuron lactate shuttle refers to a metabolic support provided by astrocytes to neurons, whereby lactate is produced by astrocytes using glucose as a precursor and provided to neurons to generate ATPs [30]. Astrocyte glucose metabolism is impaired in AD, manifesting in the form of low key glycolytic enzyme and glucose transporter (GLUT1 and GLUT3) expression [31].

The failure of this metabolism also contributes to neuronal energy loss, a decrease in synaptic plasticity, and increased susceptibility to Aβ and tau toxicity [32]. The toxic environment is further exacerbated by the impairment of mitochondrial dynamics in astrocytes, characterized by decreased oxidative phosphorylation and elevated production of ROS [33].

2.4 Astrocyte–tau interactions

A central feature of AD is tau pathology, and recent findings indicate an involvement of astrocytes in tau-related neurotoxicity [34]. Despite the role of neurons as the progenitors of pathological tau, astrocytes are capable of incorporating extracellular tau (in particular, its phosphorylated variants) via endocytosis [35]. Nonetheless, instead of completely eliminating it, the astrocytes can also facilitate tau propagation through the secretion of tau-loaded exosomes or even by transferring it to adjacent cells [36].

Besides, tau aggregation causes astrocytes to switch to a reactive phenotype (excessive expression of GFAP and secretion of pro-inflammatory cytokines, e.g., IL-1β, TNF-α), which, in turn, can also destroy neurons [37]. This reciprocal process facilitates the damage of a neuroinflammatory–tau–transmission cycle, which worsens cognitive decline in AD. Research also indicates that astrocytes could alter tau phosphorylation by affecting kinase and phosphatase activity, thereby contributing to the progression of tau pathology in AD [38, 39].

3. Microglia in Alzheimer's disease

Microglia are the primary innate immune cells of the brain; their progenitors are derived from the yolk sac, and they carry out crucial functions in immune surveillance, clearance of debris, synaptic remodeling, and tissue repair [40]. As illustrated in **Figure 3**, microglia have been shown to exhibit functional dichotomy in AD: in the early stages, they shift from protective phenotypes to chronic, detrimental activation as the disease progresses [41].

3.1 Protective roles in early disease

As shown in **Figure 3**, at the initial phases of AD, microglia are beneficial as they have been observed to recognize Aβ agglomerates via pattern recognition receptors, including Toll-like receptors, CD36, and scavenger receptors [42]. Such recognition induces a protective M2-like reaction, which entails the secretion of

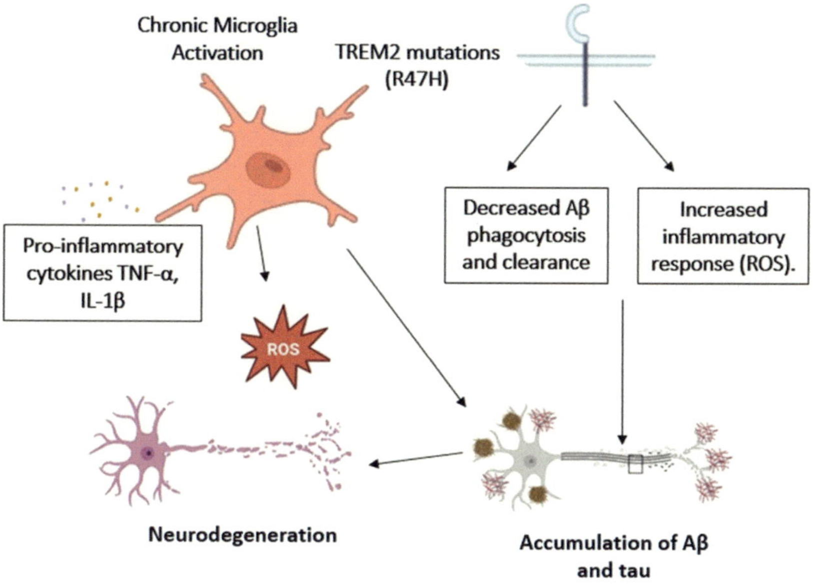

Figure 3.
Microglial dysfunction and neurodegeneration in AD.
chronic microglial activation and TREM2 mutations (R47H) reduce Aβ clearance and enhance inflammatory and oxidative stress responses, leading to Aβ and tau accumulation and progressive neurodegeneration.

anti-inflammatory cytokines such as IL-10 and TGF-β and effective phagocytosis of the Aβ [43]. Another neurotrophic factor released by microglia in this state is brain-derived neurotrophic factor, which promotes neuronal survival and synaptic activity. This period is important in inhibiting Aβ plaque formation and in initiating repair processes, yet it is normally short-lived [44].

3.2 Chronic activation and inflammation

With more severe AD pathology, continuing exposure to Aβ, oxidative damage, and damage-associated molecular patterns switches the microglial phenotype to a pro-inflammatory (M1-like) state [45]. This phenomenon results in the release of IL-1β, IL-6, TNF-α, the formation of reactive oxygen species (ROS) and nitric oxide (NO) in a neurotoxic environment, which decreases the ability of the microglia to phagocytize Aβ and degenerate cells, and increases the synaptic lesion and the death of neurons [46]. Moreover, this inflammatory signaling could also lead to hyperphosphorylation and spreading of tau, which further contributes to the progression of cognitive decline [47].

3.3 TREM2 and genetic susceptibility

The microglial surface receptor known as TREM2 (Triggering Receptor Expressed on Myeloid Cells 2) is essential for phagocytosis, Aβ binding, lipid sensing, and energy metabolism regulation [144]. TREM2 variations, especially the R47H mutation, have been found to be important genetic risk factors for late-onset AD by GWASs [48]. Signaling through TREM2 is key to the activation of a microglial subtype referred to as disease-associated microglia (DAM), the activation of which is marked by the up regulation of phagocytic and lipid metabolism genes [49]. In the AD models, loss of TREM2 causes the microglia to fail in clustering around Aβ deposition spots, phagocytosis, cholesterol homeostasis, as well as the inability to mark the DAM phenotype [50]. Furthermore, TREM2 induces microglia metabolic reprogramming, causing a shift toward glycolysis over oxidative phosphorylation, needed to provide the energetic aspect of phagocytosis and inflammatory responses [51]. The alteration of TREM2 signaling pathway consequently impairs the plasticity of microglia in the AD brain and promotes unrestricted neurodegeneration [52].

3.4 Synaptic pruning deficits

During brain development, microglia are critical in the process of synaptic pruning and in maintaining synaptic plasticity in adulthood. This is achieved through the classical complement cascade, especially the proteins C1q and C3, which mark synapses to be removed [53]. The complement, consisting of the complement receptor 3 (CR3), targets the C3-labeled synapses and causes their degradation following engulfment by the microglial cells [54].

This process of pruning is deregulated in AD. In AD mouse models, it was found that the new addition of complement oligomers enhances the expression of complement proteins and synaptic tagging, causing excessive pruning of functional synapses, specifically in the hippocampus and cortex – areas vital for memory and cognition [55]. Activation of complement is highly correlated with the diminishing of early synapses and cognition [56].

Notably, both genetic and pharmacological stimulation of complement activation abrogation in preclinical models of AD has been demonstrated to limit the loss of synapses and enhance behavior [55].

4. Oligodendrocytes and myelin dysfunction in Alzheimer's disease

Myelin dysfunction and oligodendrocytes have been found to play a significant and, in many cases, underestimated role in the pathogenesis of AD, as depicted in **Figure 4** [57]. The oligodendrocytes produce and preserve the myelin sheath, which insulates axons and enables fast transmission of nerve impulses in the CNS [58]. In AD, neuroimaging and postmortem data from multiple studies demonstrated early white matter defects, such as demyelination, thinning of myelin, and disconnection of axons, especially those related to cognitive functioning [59].

These early morphological alterations often precede atrophy of gray matter and clinical manifestations, pointing to the fact that oligodendrocyte dysfunction is not a late sequel of neuronal loss but an early and proactive element of disease pathophysiology [60]. In particular, oligodendrocytes are sensitive to oxidative stress and Aβ toxicity, both of which are extensive in AD pathology [61]. Demolition of myelin worsens the action of the axons and the synchronization among neurons, and that translates directly into cognitive deterioration [62]. The results indicate the necessity to change the focus of therapy to the preservation of the functions of, and implementation of, remyelination in order to slow or prevent the development of the disease.

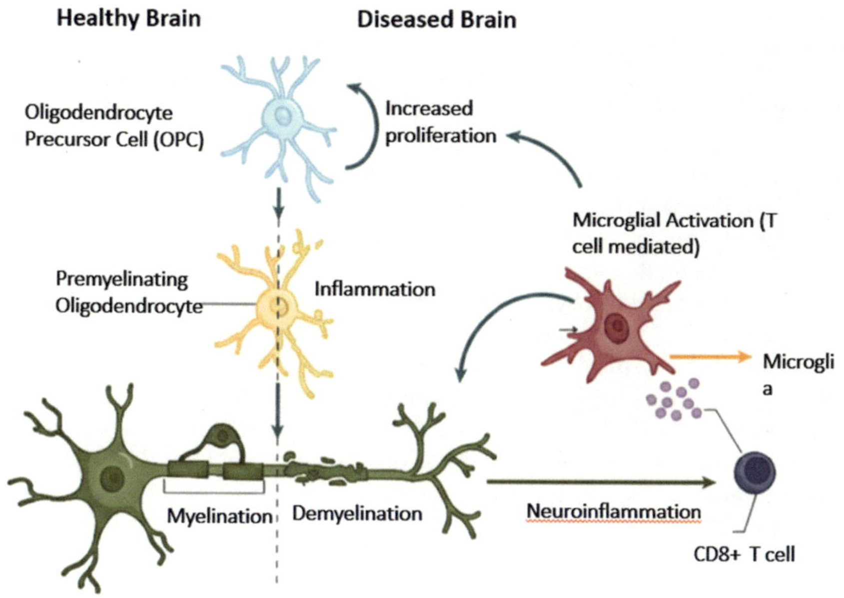

Figure 4.
Oligodendrocyte dysfunction. Normally, oligodendrocyte precursor cells (OPCs) turn into mature oligodendrocytes, which help keep myelination healthy. In some disorders, inflammation and microglial activation, which are driven by CD8⁺ T cells, interfere with OPC differentiation, resulting in excessive proliferation of OPCs and demyelination with worsening neuroinflammation.

4.1 Oxidative stress

It damages oligodendrocytes, making them vulnerable to Aβ toxicity [63]. Oligodendrocytes survive well in mild oxidative stress, but in severe oxidative stress, they exhibit high susceptibility because of high metabolic requirements and low antioxidative defense compared to other glial cells [64]. Heightened oxidative stress caused by mitochondrial dysfunction, neuroinflammation, and aggregation of Aβ in AD may lead to oligodendrocyte damage. ROS do not only harm oligodendrocyte membranes and mitochondria but also affect their performance in preserving and creating myelin sheaths [65].

In addition, oligodendrocytes are especially susceptible to amyloid-beta toxicity. It has been reported that Aβ peptides interfere with the calcium balance inside the cells, stimulate the oxidation of lipids, and induce apoptotic mechanisms in oligodendrocytes [65]. This impairs their capability to support axons, with consequent impaired white matter integrity. According to postmortem investigations, oligodendrocytes next to Aβ plaques exhibit DNA breakage and oxidative changes, suggesting their susceptibility in the AD brain [66].

4.2 Myelin breakdown

It disrupts axonal conduction and neuronal communication. These myelin sheaths play a major role in the conduction of electrical impulses along the axons. Myelin degradation in AD causes decreased conduction velocity, signal dispersion, and an inability to achieve synchronization of neurons, which is essential in memory and cognition [67]. Diffusion tensor imaging and magnetization transfer imaging studies have indicated white matter degeneration in the early stages of the disease in patients with mild cognitive impairment (MCI) and early AD, which, in some patients, occurs even before hippocampal atrophy [59].

Bartzokis (2011) put forward the myelin model of AD, that is, that the known age-dependent deterioration of myelin brings about a cascade of pathological events, including Aβ deposition and tau over-phosphorylation [66]. These regions that experience the greatest susceptibility to myelin breakdown (e.g., frontal lobes, corpus callosum) coincide with the first parts of the brain to experience cognitive impairments in AD [68]. This helps to explain that the integrity of myelin is more than a marker of the neurodegenerative changes in the disease, but also a driver. Moreover, the disintegration of myelin can be followed by the release of iron and other neurotoxins, contributing even further to the occurrence of oxidative stress and inflammation in the brain [68]. It has also been found that the loss of trophic-supporting oligodendrocytes increases the susceptibility of neurons toward degeneration [69].

4.3 OPC differentiation

Failure limits repair, leading to progressive cognitive impairment. The adult brain contains large numbers of OPCs that produce new oligodendrocytes throughout life, particularly during or after injury or demyelination. However, in AD, the differentiation of OPCs into mature myelinating oligodendrocytes is substantially impaired [70]. It has been found that Aβ oligomers and inflammatory cytokines like TNF-α and IL-1β reduce OPC proliferation and differentiation [71]. This causes impaired remyelination capacity, which complements the progressive loss of white matter integrity. Moreover, Wnt/beta-catenin and Notch signaling pathways, critical to OPC formation, have been dysregulated in AD models due to internal molecular barriers to repair [72]. The inability of OPCs to differentiate restricts endogenous repair and leads to chronic myelin deficits. Such an absence of remyelination not only derails axonal functioning but also negatively affects cognitive activities, including learning, attention, and memory [73].

5. Glial cells in prion diseases

Prion diseases are a group of transmissible and fatal neurodegenerative diseases marked by the misfolding of prion proteins (PrPSc) that spread by converting the regular cellular prion protein (PrPSc) into their diseased form [74]. This distinct self-perpetuating process causes the death of neurons, spongiform degeneration, as well as a rapid loss of cognitive and motor capabilities [75]. Glial cells, especially astrocytes, microglia, and oligodendrocytes, play a significant role in the progression and neuropathology of prion diseases, including Creutzfeldt-Jakob disease (CJD), Gerstmann-Sträussler-Scheinker syndrome (GSS), and kuru [13]. These cells, traditionally thought of as secondary responders, are now known to play an active role in prion replication, neuroinflammation, and neurodegeneration.

5.1 Astrocytes: Prion carriers and amplifiers

The most prevalent glial cells in the CNS, astrocytes, become highly reactive during the course of prion disease [76]. This increased responsiveness is known as astrogliosis and is accompanied by hypertrophy, elevated GFAP, and altered expression patterns of genes [77]. Although originally considered to be neuroprotective, reactive astrocytes may switch to a maladaptive phenotype that promotes neuroinflammation and neuronal loss [78].

It is worth noting that astrocytes are not simply passive observers to the progress of prion diseases; in fact, they are capable of intracellular replication of prions. In vitro and in vivo experiments showed that even without the involvement of cells of the nervous system, astrocytes can enhance the accumulation and spread of PrPSc [79]. This shows that astrocytes might be prion reservoirs that mediate local amplification as well as intercellular transmission of PrPSc. This activity of the astrocytes infected with prions results in inflammatory cytokines (IL-1, TNF-alpha, and IL-6), which may interfere with synaptic activity, leading to neurotoxicity [80].

Alongside retaining PrPSc, reactive astrocytes secrete a variety of pro-inflammatory cytokines, such as interleukin-1β (IL-1β), TNF-α, and IL-6, which may contribute to neurodegeneration by increasing neuronal stress and disrupting synaptic function [81]. Their protective functions, involving regulation of extracellular ions, clearing neurotransmitters, and providing metabolic support, are diminished too. This further leads to the continued degradation of the CNS microenvironment [82].

5.2 Microglia: Hyperactivation and ineffective clearance

The most familiar CNS immune cells are the microglia, and they form the initial line of defense after prion infection [83]. Activation of the microglia occurs when they detect PrPSc deposition, elicited by morphological alterations, proliferation, and immune activation through the upregulation of immune markers, that is, CD68, MHC-II, and TREM2 [84].

5.2.1 Prolonged inflammation

Prolonged inflammation leads to a cytokine cascade that worsens neuronal loss [85]. Microglial activation is protective at the early stage, as it attempts to phagocytose prion-infected debris and ensure homeostasis; however, in chronic prion disease, this becomes maladaptive [86]. Microglia release prolonged expression of pro-inflammatory mediators, such as TNF-α, IL-1β, and interferon-gamma (IFN-γ), triggering a cytokine storm that disrupts neuron-glia homeostasis and accelerates neurodegeneration [87].

5.2.2 Inefficient phagocytosis

Despite microglial activation, they exhibit limited capacity to clear PrPSc, resisting lysosomal degradation, which results in the accumulation of this misfolded prion protein within microglial cells, which, in turn, contributes to their functional impairment [88]. Microglial activation in the presence of PrPSc leads to the release of ROS and nitric oxide (NO), which are ineffective against the pathogenic protein but contribute to oxidative injury of surrounding neural cells, thereby exacerbating the spongiform degeneration hallmarking prion pathology [89].

This unproductive clearance and persistent oxidative stress generate a negative feedback loop where microglial activation continues, increases neuron injury, and leads to the driven spread of prion diseases [90].

5.2.3 ROS and NO release

Activated microglia secrete ROS and nitric oxide (NO), which are toxic when excessive [91]. These produced molecules damage neuronal membranes, interfere with the functioning of mitochondria, and also increase lipid peroxidation, leading to the characteristic features of vacuolation and spongiform alterations in prion-affected brains [92]. Preventing microglial activation or minimizing the presence of oxidative stress has demonstrated a slowing of disease progression in experimental models, where excessive microglial activation is destructive [93].

5.3 Oligodendrocyte involvement

Oligodendrocytes, the myelinating glial cells of the CNS, play a vital role in axonal integrity, signal conduction, and cellular metabolism [94]. Their contribution to prion diseases is less well-defined than that of astrocytes and microglia, but indirect evidence suggests they are markedly affected [95]. Although the outright direct infection of oligodendrocytes by prions has not been clearly demonstrated, the inflammatory and oxidative conditions of prion disorders are most likely affecting the performance and survival of oligodendrocytes [96]. TNF-alpha and IFN-gamma cytokines are cytotoxic to OPCs, impede their maturation, and restrict their ability to engage in remyelination [97].

6. Therapeutic strategies targeting glial dysfunction

In recent years, it has become clear that glial dysfunction plays an important role in the onset and development of neurodegenerative disorders such as AD and prion disease [98]. There is a considerable shift toward focusing on glial activity modulation in therapy, as an increasing amount of evidence has attributed the role of glial cells, especially astrocytes and microglia, in driving the course of the disease. Disruption of glial cells plays a major role in chronic neuroinflammation, oxidative stress, and neuroglia injury. Therefore, targeting glial cells is a very attractive tactic to stop or reverse neurodegeneration [99].

6.1 Anti-inflammatory agents

Neurodegenerative disorders are characterized by chronic neuroinflammation, which is facilitated by activated glial cells. Regulation of such an inflammatory response through the injection of pharmacological agents may provide a possible avenue to reduce neuronal damage and enhance clinical outcomes [100].

6.1.1 NSAIDs and IL-1β antagonists

The most studied compounds in modulating glial inflammation include non-steroidal anti-inflammatory drugs (NSAIDs), such as ibuprofen, naproxen, and indomethacin. These medicines mainly restrain cyclooxygenase (COX)-1 and COX-2 enzymes, which synthesize prostaglandins – important agents of inflammation. COX-2 in the CNS is upregulated in activated microglia and leads to neurodegenerative cascades by increasing oxidative stress and excitotoxicity [101].

Transgenic mouse models of AD have been used in preclinical trials, proving that chronic treatment with NSAIDs inhibits microglial activation, plaque load, and neuronal loss [102]. It was shown, in particular, that ibuprofen decreased the expression of IL-1beta and TNF-alpha and enhanced cognitive performance in the animal models of AD [55, 103]. The human experiments, however, are contradicted in terms of the clinical trials conducted so far. The ADAPT trial (Alzheimer Disease Anti-inflammatory Prevention Trial) has not demonstrated any protective role of naproxen or celecoxib against dementia among patients with MCIs, and some NSAIDs have been reported to have cardiovascular risks [104]. This has diverted the focus to more specific cytokine inhibitory strategies, that is, IL-1 block antagonists.

Activated microglia produce an extremely strong pro-inflammatory cytokine, IL-1β [105]. It enhances the activation of astrocytes, impairs synaptic plasticity, and increases the neuroinflammatory loop. Clinical use of Anakinra, a recombinant IL-1 receptor antagonist (IL-1 Ra), has been observed in autoimmune diseases such as rheumatoid arthritis. In neurodegenerative models, the administration of IL-1 Ra suppressed the activation of glial cells, the accumulation of amyloid, and the phosphorylation of tau [106].

Furthermore, higher concentrations of IL-1 in the cerebrospinal fluid (CSF) have been linked to both the course of AD and the prion diseases, further demonstrating its therapeutic potential as a target [107, 108].

6.2 Microglia-targeted therapies

Microglia are the innate immune units of the CNS, which have a dual role in neurodegenerative diseases [109]. In homeostatic states, they mediate synaptic pruning, clearance, and neurotrophic support. However, when chronic microglial activation is present in pathologies such as AD and prion disorders, neuroinflammation, synaptic dysfunction, and neuronal loss occur [110]. Microglia have since then become a significant target in therapy. The two key pathways that are being investigated are TREM2 signaling (as it promotes positive microglial activities) and CSF1R (as it limits excessive or pathological proliferation of microglia) [9].

6.2.1 TREM2 agonists to enhance phagocytosis

Microglia have a particular receptor called triggering receptor expressed on myeloid cells 2 (TREM2) that controls phagocytosis, lipid metabolism, and inflammatory response. Mutations causing loss of function in the TREM2 gene show the protective effect of this gene and predispose people to AD [111, 112]. TREM2 mediates the switch of microglia into a phenotype of their newly understood form, the so-called disease-associated-microglia (DAM), which intensively phagocytose Aβ and apoptotic debris [113].

The treatment interventions (based on TREM2 agonist antibodies) are intended to enhance the effectiveness of microglia. The most prominent example is a monoclonal antibody, AL002 developed by Alector and licensed to AbbVie. Preclinical research demonstrated that AL002 improved TREM2 signaling, amplified microglial aggregation at plaques, lowered amyloid pathology, and maintained synaptic integrity [114].

6.2.2 CSF1R inhibitors to modulate microglial proliferation

Colony-stimulating factor 1 receptor (CSF1R) is a tyrosine kinase receptor important for the survival, proliferation, and differentiation of microglia [115]. Persistent activation or overexpression of CSF1R is associated with neurotoxicity, hyper-microgliosis, and transmission of neurodegeneration, which is linked to the pathology [116, 117].

CSF1R inhibition causes depletion or proliferation arrest in microglia, resulting in decreased neuroinflammation and secondary damage [118]. In mice carrying AD, treatment with a CSF1R inhibitor leads to decreased microgliosis related to plaque parenchyma, reduced cytokines of immune response, and neural protection and functional neurorestoration [119].

While reduction at later stages produced less benefit and ran the risk of compromising synaptic support, a study showed that early and persistent microglial ablation with a CSF1R inhibitor in 5xFAD Alzheimer's mice decreased amyloid plaque growth, neuronal loss, and enhanced memory [120]. In this way, partial or temporary inhibition is now considered a moderate therapy. The same effects have been observed in prion diseases with inhibition of CSF1R, where elimination of microglia slowed the progression of the disease, decreased levels of PrPSc, and reduced neuronal vacuolation [121]. This supports the hypothesis that proliferative pathogenic microglia contribute to neurodegeneration outside amyloid pathology-based diseases.

6.3 Astrocyte modulators

Astrocytes are key factors in preserving CNS homeostasis by regulating neurotransmitter diffusion, providing support to the BBB, and adjusting synaptic dynamics [89]. However, reactive astrogliosis of the astrocytes is a transformation that occurs during neurodegeneration, characterized by morphological distortion, expression of inflammatory genes, and the loss of homeostatic mechanisms [45]. Treatments that either rejuvenate astrocytes or inhibit pathological reactivity are emerging as potential therapies for AD and prion diseases.

6.3.1 Compounds that upregulate EAAT2 expression

Excitatory amino acid transporter 2 (EAAT2), or more commonly GLT-1 in rodents, removes more than 90% of extracellular glutamate in the CNS and thus eliminates excitatory toxicity – a major causative component of neurodegeneration in various conditions such as AD or amyotrophic lateral sclerosis (ALS). EAAT2 is mostly astroglial, and its reduction is usually reported in neurodegenerative pathologies [122].

The EAAT2-upregulating therapies can work in terms of affecting a restoration of glutamate homeostasis and the prevention of cell death. Among its compounds is the following notable compound:

6.3.1.1 Ceftriaxone

It is a β-lactam antibiotic with a high effect on EAAT2 transcription. Ceftriaxone also increased EAAT2 in vivo and in vitro models, thereby enhancing motor performance and survival in ALS mice. Ceftriaxone therapy in AD models attenuated amyloid pathology and enhanced cognition [122, 123].

6.3.1.2 MS-153 and LDN/OSU-0212320

These are small molecules that are known to stimulate EAAT2 promoter, resulting in either the upregulation of EAAT2 and the removal of neurodegenerative glutamate toxicity in experimental models [124, 125].

In animal models, adeno-associated viral vectors-based gene therapy strategies to express EAAT2 by overexpression appear promising and have been shown to ameliorate neurodegeneration and inflammation [126].

6.3.2 Targeting JAK/STAT signaling in reactive astrogliosis

A significant pathway of the signaling cascade that is associated with reactive astrogliosis is the Janus kinase/signal transducer and activator of transcription (JAK/STAT) pathway [127]. Neurodegenerative diseases are accompanied by long-term activation of the JAK/STAT3 signaling pathway in astrocytes, with a loss of favorable neuroprotective properties and a shift to more neurotoxic behavior [128]. Therefore, the inhibition of maladaptive astrogliosis through JAK/STAT signaling suppression is under development.

6.3.2.1 STAT3 conditional knockout

Conditional knockout of STAT3 in AD mouse models with astrocyte-specific deletion leads to a reduction in astrocyte reactivity and better survival of neurons, along with a smaller number of plaques [129].

6.3.2.2 WP1066 and AG490

These are small molecular inhibitors of JAK2/STAT3 signaling, and with them, astrogliosis and production of cytokines are decreased, resulting in neuroprotection in models of prion disease and traumatic brain injury [130, 131].

Ciliary neurotrophic factor (CNTF): Although CNTF can stimulate the JAK/STAT signaling pathway, low doses or transient activation could reprogram astrocytes toward a pro-protective phenotype, and thus moderate, rather than complete, inhibition of this pathway may be desirable at certain stages of disease progression [128].

6.4 Gene and cell-based therapies

The use of genes and cells is gaining traction in the management of neurodegenerative diseases, particularly those that are glia-prominent, especially AD and prion diseases [132]. The strategies aim to reverse genetic risk factors or remove dysfunctional glia by replacing them with new, healthy, functional cells, which may ultimately stop or even roll back the disease process [133].

6.4.1 CRISPR-Cas9 correction of glial risk alleles (e.g., TREM2, APOE4)

Genetic variants in glia-expressed genes, that is, APOE and TREM2, are found to be predominantly linked with increased chances of AD and neurodegenerative disorders [134]. CRISPR-Cas9 genome editing has made it possible to target such risk alleles at their source and accomplish this in a cell-type-specific fashion.

6.4.1.1 Correction of APOE4

The strongest risk factor in genetic terms for sporadic AD was found to be the APOE4 allele, which is expressed mainly in astrocytes and, more weakly, in microglia. APOE4 promotes poor clearance of Aβ, enhances inflammation, and compounds damage to the BBB. Conversion of APOE4-associated AD patient iPSC-derived astrocytes to an APOE3 isoform with a neutral phenotype using CRISPR-Cas9 regulated cholesterol metabolism, decreased the secretion of Aβ, and enhanced the supporting features of astrocytes [135]. Base editing technologies have demonstrated the possibility of APOE4 to APOE3 in mouse brains both in vitro and in vivo, which decreases neuroinflammation and Aβ load [136].

6.4.1.2 The correction of TREM2

TREM2 is a receptor expressed in microglial cells that mediates phagocytosis and inflammatory responses, and pathogenic forms of TREM2 favor AD by dysregulating microglial responses to Aβ. In a 2021 study, the R47H mutation in microglia derived from induced pluripotent stem cells (iPSCs) was corrected with the help of CRISPR-Cas9. In chimeric mouse models and in vitro, gene-corrected microglia exhibited restored phagocytic ability, a correct metabolic profile, and a better response to plaques [137, 138]

6.4.2 Transplantation of healthy glial progenitors or stem-cell-derived astrocytes

The next potentially promising direction in the transplantation of healthy glial progenitors or astrocytes produced by pluripotent stem cells is glial-targeted therapy [139]. This is aimed at replacing dysfunctional glia and re-establishing the neuroprotective effects of the diseased CNS.

6.4.2.1 Astrocyte transplantation

Transplantation of human embryonic stem-cell-derived astrocytes (hESCs) or induced pluripotent stem-cell-derived astrocytes (iPSCs) into AD and ALS mouse models is possible. This population of astrocytes is characterized by infiltration into the host tissue, stabilization of neurons, absorption of the extracellular form of glutamate, as well as dampening of inflammation [140]. Transplantation of iPSC-derived astrocytes decreased Aβ burden, ameliorated synaptic plasticity, and corrected cognitive impairment in an AD model mouse [141].

6.4.2.2 Transplantation of glial progenitor

Glial progenitor cells (GPCs), which have the potential to differentiate into both astrocytes and oligodendrocytes, are another prospective cellular therapy. GPCs remyelinate axons, enhance behavioral therapies, reduce neuroinflammation, and improve outcomes in leukodystrophy and demyelination in mouse models [142, 143]. Although research on prion diseases is scarce, due to the dense astro-glial/oligo-glial participation in the pathogenesis, the possibility of alleviating functional loss by substituting these cells exists.

7. Conclusion

Alzheimer's disease has long been described primarily in terms of neuronal dysfunction and the pathogenic accumulations of amyloid-beta and tau, but it is now generally regarded as a disease involving the complex interplay among all components of the cells in the CNS. These include the glial cells, which play an instrumental role in the onset and progression of neurodegenerative processes, and encompass astrocytes, microglia, and oligodendrocytes. Astrocytes, once thought to be passive support cells, are now recognized as active modulators of neuroinflammation and neurotransmission. Their reactive phenotype in AD not only disrupts glutamate homeostasis and fuel supply but also contributes to amyloid and tau pathology. Similarly, microglia exhibit highly variable functional roles, where their initial protective response to amyloid-beta is overshadowed by long-term pro-inflammatory activation, which causes neuronal damage, loss of synaptic sites due to complement activity, and defective clearance processes, particularly in carriers of hereditary mutations such as TREM2. Meanwhile, oligodendrocytes and their precursors, which are often overlooked, are also significantly affected by AD pathology. Abnormal neural communication arises from oxidative stress, defective OPC differentiation, and the degeneration of myelin, which exacerbates cognitive decline. These white matter changes are becoming increasingly apparent at early stages in imaging tests and can be detected before the onset of classic AD symptoms. In combination, the malfunction of glial cells can amplify the classical symptomatic pathology of AD and, additionally, represents a therapeutically untapped area of interest. Understanding and modulating glial-specific therapies (e.g., enhancing astrocytic clearance, reprogramming or remodeling microglia, and repairing oligodendrocytes) is another promising avenue for disease-modifying innovations. A potential new perspective on the so-called gliocentric pathology in AD prompts a redefinition of therapeutic approaches to account for the complex and essential functions of glial cells in maintaining CNS homeostasis.

Conflict of Interest

The authors declare no conflict of interest.

Author details

Saima Zafar[1,2,3*], Urwah Rasheed[1,2] and Inga Zerr[1,2]

1 Department of Neurology, University Medical Center, Georg-August Universitäts Göttingen, Göttingen, Germany

2 German Center for Neurodegenerative Diseases (DZNE), Göttingen, Germany

3 Biomedical Engineering and Sciences Department, School of Mechanical and Manufacturing Engineering (SMME), National University of Sciences and Technology (NUST), Islamabad, Pakistan

*Address all correspondence to: sz_awaan@yahoo.com

References

[1] Jellinger KA. Basic mechanisms of neurodegeneration: A critical update. Journal of Cellular and Molecular Medicine. 2010;**14**(3):457–487. DOI: 10.1111/j.1582-4934.2010.01010.x

[2] Stobart JL, Anderson CM. Multifunctional role of astrocytes as gatekeepers of neuronal energy supply. Frontiers in Cellular Neuroscience. 2013;**7**:38. DOI: 10.3389/fncel.2013.00038

[3] Kwon HS, Koh SH. Neuroinflammation in neurodegenerative disorders: The roles of microglia and astrocytes. Translational Neurodegeneration. 2020;**9**:42. DOI: 10.1186/s40035-020-00221-2

[4] Müller L, Di Benedetto S. Neuroimmune crosstalk in chronic neuroinflammation: Microglial interactions and immune modulation. Frontiers in Cellular Neuroscience. 2025;**19**:1575022

[5] Quan L, Uyeda A, Muramatsu R. Central nervous system regeneration: The roles of glial cells in the potential molecular mechanism underlying remyelination. Inflammation and Regeneration. 2022;**42**(1):7. DOI: 10.1186/s41232-022-00193-y

[6] Colonna M, Butovsky O. Microglia function in the central nervous system during health and neurodegeneration. Annual Review of Immunology. 2017;**35**:441–468. DOI: 10.1146/annurev-immunol-051116-052358

[7] Verkhratsky A, Butt A, Li B, et al. Astrocytes in human central nervous system diseases: A frontier for new therapies. Signal Transduction and Targeted Therapy. 2023;**8**:396

[8] Escartin C, Galea E, Lakatos A, et al. Reactive astrocyte nomenclature, definitions, and future directions. Nature Neuroscience. 2021;**24**:312–325

[9] Villegas-Llerena C, Phillips A, Garcia-Reitboeck P, Hardy J, Pocock JM. Microglial genes regulating neuroinflammation in the progression of Alzheimer's disease. Current Opinion in Neurobiology. 2016;**36**:74–81. DOI: 10.1016/j.conb.2015.10.004

[10] Liddelow S, Guttenplan K, Clarke L, et al. Neurotoxic reactive astrocytes are induced by activated microglia. Nature. 2017;**541**:481–487

[11] Öztürk MM, Emgård J, García-Revilla J, Fernández-Calle R, Yang Y, Deierborg T, Roos TT. The role of microglia in the prion-like transmission of protein aggregates in neurodegeneration. Brain Communications. 2025;7(2):fcaf087. DOI: 10.1093/braincomms/fcaf087

[12] Bradford BM, McGuire LI, Hume DA, Pridans C, Mabbott NA. Microglia deficiency accelerates prion disease but does not enhance prion accumulation in the brain. Glia. 2022;**70**(11):2169–2187. DOI: 10.1002/glia.24244

[13] Smethurst P, Franklin H, Clarke BE, Sidle K, Patani R. The role of astrocytes in prion-like mechanisms of neurodegeneration. Brain. 2022;**145**(1):17–26. DOI: 10.1093/brain/awab366

[14] Ising C, Venegas C, Zhang S, et al. NLRP3 inflammasome activation drives

tau pathology. Nature. 2019;**575**: 669–673

[15] Condello C, Yuan P, Neuroprotection GJM-M. TREM2, and Alzheimer's disease: Evidence from optical imaging. Biological Psychiatry. 2018;**83**(4):377–387. DOI: 10.1016/j.biopsych.2017.10.007

[16] Gao C, Jiang J, Tan Y, et al. Microglia in neurodegenerative diseases: Mechanism and potential therapeutic targets. Signal Transduction and Targeted Therapy. 2023;**8**:359

[17] Lawal O, Ulloa Severino FP, Eroglu C. The role of astrocyte structural plasticity in regulating neural circuit function and behavior. Glia. 2022;**70**(8):1467–1483. DOI: 10.1002/glia.24191

[18] Verkhratsky A, Nedergaard M. Physiology of astroglia. Physiological Reviews. 2018;**98**(1):239–389. DOI: 10.1152/physrev.00042.2016

[19] Liddelow SA, Barres BA. Reactive astrocytes: Production, function, and therapeutic potential. Immunity. 2017;**46**(6):957–967

[20] Wyss-Coray T, Loike J, Brionne T, *et al.* Adult mouse astrocytes degrade amyloid-β in vitro and in situ. Nature Medicine. 2003;**9**:453–457

[21] Ries M, Sastre M. Mechanisms of Aβ clearance and degradation by glial cells. Frontiers in Aging Neuroscience. 2016;**8**:160

[22] Heneka MT, Carson MJ, El Khoury J, Landreth GE, Brosseron F, Feinstein DL, Kummer MP et al. Neuroinflammation in Alzheimer's disease. The Lancet Neurology. 2015;**14**(4):388–405

[23] Azargoonjahromi A. The duality of amyloid-β: Its role in normal and Alzheimer's disease states. Molecular Brain. 2024;**17**(1):44. DOI: 10.1186/s13041-024-01118-1

[24] Habib N, McCabe C, Medina S, et al. Disease-associated astrocytes in Alzheimer's disease and aging. Nature Neuroscience. 2020;**23**:701–706

[25] Mahmoud S, Gharagozloo M, Simard C, Gris D. Astrocytes maintain glutamate homeostasis in the CNS by controlling the balance between glutamate uptake and release. Cells. 2019;**8**(2):184. DOI: 10.3390/cells8020184

[26] Takahashi K, Foster JB, Lin CL. Glutamate transporter EAAT2: Regulation, function, and potential as a therapeutic target for neurological and psychiatric disease. Cellular and Molecular Life Sciences. 2015;**72**(18):3489–3506. DOI: 10.1007/s00018-015-1937-8

[27] Dong XX, Wang Y, ZH Q. Molecular mechanisms of excitotoxicity and their relevance to pathogenesis of neurodegenerative diseases. Acta Pharmacologica Sinica. 2009;**30**(4):379–387. DOI: 10.1038/aps.2009.24

[28] Mason S. Lactate shuttles in neuroenergetics—homeostasis, allostasis and beyond. Frontiers in Neuroscience. 2017;**11**:43

[29] Beard E, Lengacher S, Dias S, Magistretti PJ, Finsterwald C. Astrocytes as key regulators of brain energy metabolism: New therapeutic perspectives. Frontiers in Physiology. 2022;**12**:825816

[30] Kim Y, Dube SE, Park CB. Brain energy homeostasis: The evolution of

the astrocyte-neuron lactate shuttle hypothesis. The Korean Journal of Physiology & Pharmacology. 2025;**29**(1):1–8. DOI: 10.4196/kjpp.24.388

[31] Raut S, Bhalerao A, Powers M, Gonzalez M, Mancuso S, Cucullo L. Hypometabolism, Alzheimer's disease, and possible therapeutic targets: An overview. Cells. 2023;**12**(16):2019. DOI: 10.3390/cells12162019

[32] Yuan Y, Zhao G, Zhao Y. Dysregulation of energy metabolism in Alzheimer's disease. Journal of Neurology. 2024;**272**(1):2. DOI: 10.1007/s00415-024-12800-8

[33] Meng K, Jia H, Hou X, Zhu Z, Lu Y, Feng Y, Feng J, Xia Y, Tan R, Cui F, Yuan J. Mitochondrial dysfunction in neurodegenerative diseases: Mechanisms and corresponding therapeutic strategies. Biomedicines. 2025;**13**(2):327. DOI: 10.3390/biomedicines13020327

[34] Chen Y, Yu Y. Tau and neuroinflammation in Alzheimer's disease: Interplay mechanisms and clinical translation. Journal of Neuroinflammation. 2023;**20**:165. DOI: 10.1186/s12974-023-02853-3

[35] Brunello CA, Merezhko M, Uronen RL, Huttunen HJ. Mechanisms of secretion and spreading of pathological tau protein. Cellular and Molecular Life Sciences. 2020;**77**(9):1721–1744. DOI: 10.1007/s00018-019-03349-1

[36] Deng Q, Wu C, Parker E, Liu TC, Duan R, Yang L. Microglia and astrocytes in Alzheimer's disease: Significance and summary of recent advances. Aging and Disease. 2024;**15**(4):1537–1564. DOI: 10.14336/AD.2023.0907

[37] Han J, Zhang Z, Zhang P, Yu Q, Cheng Q, Lu Z, Zong S. The roles of microglia and astrocytes in neuroinflammation of Alzheimer's disease. Frontiers in Neuroscience. 2025;**19**:1575453. DOI: 10.3389/fnins.2025.1575453

[38] Garwood CJ, Pooler AM, Atherton J, Hanger DP, Noble W. Astrocytes are important mediators of Aβ-induced neurotoxicity and tau phosphorylation in primary culture. Cell Death & Disease. 2011;**2**(6):e167. DOI: 10.1038/cddis.2011.50

[39] Bellaver B, Povala G, Ferreira PC, Ferrari-Souza JP, Leffa DT, Lussier FZ, Pascoal TA et al. Astrocyte reactivity influences amyloid-β effects on tau pathology in preclinical Alzheimer's disease. Nature Medicine. 2023;**29**(7):1775–1781

[40] Casali BT, Reed-Geaghan EG. Microglial function and regulation during development, homeostasis and Alzheimer's disease. Cells. 2021;**10**(4):957. DOI: 10.3390/cells10040957

[41] Valiukas Z, Tangalakis K, Apostolopoulos V, Feehan J. Microglial activation states and their implications for Alzheimer's disease. The Journal of Prevention of Alzheimer's Disease. 2025;**100013**

[42] Jin JJ, Kim HD, Maxwell JA, Li L, Fukuchi KI. Toll-like receptor 4-dependent upregulation of cytokines in a transgenic mouse model of Alzheimer's disease. Journal of Neuroinflammation. 2008;**5**:1–10

[43] Cherry JD, Olschowka JA, O'Banion MK. Neuroinflammation and M2 microglia: The good, the bad, and the inflamed. Journal of Neuroinflammation.

2014;**11**:98. DOI: 10.1186/1742-2094-11-98

[44] Trang T, Beggs S, Salter MW. Brain-derived neurotrophic factor from microglia: A molecular substrate for neuropathic pain. Neuron Glia Biology. 2011;7(1):99–108. DOI: 10.1017/S1740925X12000087

[45] Ghimire A, Rehman SA, Subhani A, Khan MA, Rahman Z, Iqubal MK, Iqubal A. Mechanism of microglia-mediated neuroinflammation, associated cognitive dysfunction, and therapeutic updates in Alzheimer's disease. hLife. 2025;**3**:64–81

[46] Cai Y, Liu J, Wang B, Sun M, Yang H. Microglia in the neuroinflammatory pathogenesis of Alzheimer's disease and related therapeutic targets. Frontiers in Immunology. 2022;**13**:856376. DOI: 10.3389/fimmu.2022.856376

[47] Dias D, Socodato R. Beyond amyloid and tau: The critical role of microglia in Alzheimer's disease therapeutics. Biomedicines. 2025;**13**(2):279. DOI: 10.3390/biomedicines13020279

[48] Yaghmoor F, Noorsaeed A, Alsaggaf S, Aljohani W, Scholtzova H, Boutajangout A, Wisniewski T. The role of TREM2 in Alzheimer's disease and other neurological disorders. Journal of Alzheimer's Disease & Parkinsonism. 2014;**4**(5):160. DOI: 10.4172/2161-0460.1000160

[49] Cantoni C, Bollman B, Licastro D, Xie M, Mikesell R, Schmidt R, Yuede CM, Galimberti D, Olivecrona G, Klein RS, Cross AH, Otero K, Piccio L. TREM2 regulates microglial cell activation in response to demyelination in vivo. Acta Neuropathologica. 2015;**129**(3):429–447. DOI: 10.1007/s00401-015-1388-1

[50] Zhang L, Xiang X, Li Y, Bu G, Chen XF. TREM2 and sTREM2 in Alzheimer's disease: From mechanisms to therapies. Molecular Neurodegeneration. 2025;**20**(1):43. DOI: 10.1186/s13024-025-00834-z

[51] Huang Q, Wang Y, Chen S, Liang F. Glycometabolic reprogramming of microglia in neurodegenerative diseases: Insights from neuroinflammation. Aging and Disease. 2024;**15**(3):1155–1175. DOI: 10.14336/AD.2023.0807

[52] Shi Q, Gutierrez RA, Bhat MA. Microglia, Trem2, and neurodegeneration. The Neuroscientist: A Review Journal Bringing Neurobiology, Neurology and Psychiatry. 2025;**31**(2):159–176. DOI: 10.1177/10738584241254118

[53] Wu Y, Dissing-Olesen L, MacVicar BA, Stevens B. Microglia: dynamic mediators of synapse development and plasticity. Trends in Immunology. 2015;**36**(10):605–613. DOI: 10.1016/j.it.2015.08.008

[54] Paolicelli RC, Ferretti MT. Function and dysfunction of microglia during brain development: Consequences for synapses and neural circuits. Frontiers in Synaptic Neuroscience. 2017;**9**:9. DOI: 10.3389/fnsyn.2017.00009

[55] Shi Q, Chowdhury S, Ma R, Le KX, Hong S, Caldarone BJ, Stevens B, Lemere CA. Complement C3 deficiency protects against neurodegeneration in aged plaque-rich APP/PS1 mice. Science Translational Medicine. 2017;**9**(392):eaaf6295. DOI: 10.1126/scitranslmed.aaf6295

[56] Spurrier J, Nicholson L, Fang XT, Stoner AJ, Toyonaga T, Holden D, Siegert TR, Laird W, Allnutt MA, Chiasseu M, Brody AH, Takahashi H, Nies SH, Pérez-Cañamás A, Sadasivam P, Lee S, Li S, Zhang L, Huang YH, Carson RE, Strittmatter SM. Reversal of synapse loss in Alzheimer mouse models by targeting mGluR5 to prevent synaptic tagging by C1Q. Science Translational Medicine. 2022;**14**(647):eabi8593. DOI: 10.1126/scitranslmed.abi8593

[57] Badina AM, Ceyzériat K, Amossé Q, Tresh A, Abjean L, Guénat L, Tournier BB, et al. Non-linear microglial, inflammatory and oligodendrocyte dynamics across stages of Alzheimer's disease. Neurobiology of Disease. 2025;**106950**

[58] Simons M, Nave KA. Oligodendrocytes: Myelination and axonal support. Cold Spring Harbor Perspectives in Biology. 2015;**8**(1): a020479. DOI: 10.1101/cshperspect.a020479

[59] Zhou J, Zhang P, Zhang B, Kong Y. White matter damage in Alzheimer's disease: Contribution of oligodendrocytes. Current Alzheimer Research. 2022;**19**(9):629–640. DOI: 10.2174/1567205020666221021115321

[60] Nasrabady SE, Rizvi B, Goldman JE, *et al.* White matter changes in Alzheimer's disease: A focus on myelin and oligodendrocytes. Acta Neuropathologica Communications. 2018;**6**(22). DOI: 10.1186/s40478-018-0515-3

[61] Desai MK, Mastrangelo MA, Ryan DA, Sudol KL, Narrow WC, Bowers WJ. Early oligodendrocyte/myelin pathology in Alzheimer's disease mice constitutes a novel therapeutic target. The American Journal of Pathology. 2010;**177**(3):1422–1435. DOI: 10.2353/ajpath.2010.100087

[62] Khelfaoui H, Ibaceta-Gonzalez C, Angulo MC. Functional myelin in cognition and neurodevelopmental disorders. Cellular and Molecular Life Sciences. 2024;**81**(1):181. DOI: 10.1007/s00018-024-05222-2

[63] Roth AD, Ramírez G, Alarcón R, Von Bernhardi R. Oligodendrocytes damage in Alzheimer's disease: Beta amyloid toxicity and inflammation. Biological Research. 2005;**38**(4):381–387

[64] Jy K, JH K, Yd K, Seo JH. High vulnerability of oligodendrocytes to oxidative stress induced by ultrafine urban particles. Antioxidants (Basel). 2020;**10**(1):4. DOI: 10.3390/antiox10010004

[65] Spaas J, van Veggel L, Schepers M, Tiane A, van Horssen J, Wilson 3rd DM, Moya PR, Piccart E, Hellings N, Eijnde BO, Derave W, Schreiber R, Vanmierlo T. Oxidative stress and impaired oligodendrocyte precursor cell differentiation in neurological disorders. Cellular and Molecular Life Sciences. 2021;**78**(10):4615–4637. DOI: 10.1007/s00018-021-03802-0

[66] Bartzokis G. Alzheimer's disease as homeostatic responses to age-related myelin breakdown. Neurobiology of Aging. 2011;**32**(8):1341–1371

[67] Papuć E, Rejdak K. The role of myelin damage in Alzheimer's disease pathology. Archives of Medical Science. 2018;**16**(2):345–351. DOI: 10.5114/aoms.2018.76863

[68] Bartzokis G, Lu PH, Mintz J. Human brain myelination and amyloid beta deposition in Alzheimer's disease.

Alzheimer's & Dementia: The Journal of the Alzheimer's Association. 2007;**3**(2):122–125. DOI: 10.1016/j.jalz.2007.01.019

[69] Maitre M, Jeltsch-David H, Okechukwu NG, et al. Myelin in Alzheimer's disease: Culprit or bystander? Acta Neuropathologica Communications. 2023;**11**(56). DOI: 10.1186/s40478-023-01554-5

[70] El Waly B, Macchi M, Cayre M, Durbec P. Oligodendrogenesis in the normal and pathological central nervous system. Frontiers in Neuroscience. 2014;**8**:145. DOI: 10.3389/fnins.2014.00145

[71] Beiter RM, Raghavan TP, Suchocki O, Ennerfelt HE, Rivet-Noor CR, Merchak AR, Phillips JL, Bathe T, Lukens JR, Prokop S, Dupree JL, Gaultier A. Oligomeric amyloid beta prevents myelination in a clusterin-dependent manner. Research Square. 2024; DOI: 10.21203/rs.3.rs-4415143/v1. rs.3.rs-4415143

[72] Zou P, Wu C, Liu TC, Duan R, Yang L. Oligodendrocyte progenitor cells in Alzheimer's disease: From physiology to pathology. Translational Neurodegeneration. 2023;**12**(1):52. DOI: 10.1186/s40035-023-00385-7

[73] Zveik O, Rechtman A, Ganz T, Vaknin-Dembinsky A. The interplay of inflammation and remyelination: Rethinking MS treatment with a focus on oligodendrocyte progenitor cells. Molecular Neurodegeneration. 2024;**19**(1):53. DOI: 10.1186/s13024-024-00742-8

[74] Prusiner SB, Prions. Proceedings of the National Academy of Sciences of the United States of America. 1998;**95**(23):13363–13383. DOI: 10.1073/pnas.95.23.13363

[75] Hughes D, Halliday M. What is our current understanding of PrP^{Sc}-associated neurotoxicity and its molecular underpinnings? Pathogens (Basel, Switzerland). 2017;**6**(4):63. DOI: 10.3390/pathogens6040063

[76] Hay A, Popichak K, Moreno J, Zabel M. The role of glial cells in neurobiology and prion neuropathology. Cells. 2024;**13**(10):832. DOI: 10.3390/cells13100832

[77] Lawrence JM, Schardien K, Wigdahl B, Nonnemacher MR. Roles of neuropathology-associated reactive astrocytes: A systematic review. Acta Neuropathologica Communications. 2023;**11**(1):42. DOI: 10.1186/s40478-023-01526-9

[78] Ding ZB, Song LJ, Wang Q, Kumar G, Yan YQ, Ma CG. Astrocytes: A double-edged sword in neurodegenerative diseases. Neural Regeneration Research. 2021;**16**(9):1702–1710. DOI: 10.4103/1673-5374.306064

[79] Tahir W, Thapa S, Schatzl HM. Astrocyte in prion disease: A double-edged sword. Neural Regeneration Research. 2022;**17**(8):1659–1665. DOI: 10.4103/1673-5374.332202

[80] Lakkaraju AKK, Sorce S, Senatore A, Nuvolone M, Guo J, Schwarz P, Moos R, Pelczar P, Aguzzi A. Glial activation in prion diseases is selectively triggered by neuronal PrPSc. Brain Pathology (Zurich, Switzerland). 2022;**32**(5):e13056. DOI: 10.1111/bpa.13056

[81] Lim GP, Yang F, Chu T, Chen P, Beech W, Teter B, Tran T, Ubeda O, Ashe KH, Frautschy SA, Cole GM. Ibuprofen suppresses plaque pathology

and inflammation in a mouse model for Alzheimer's disease. The Journal of Neuroscience. 2000;**20**(15):5709–5714. DOI: 10.1523/JNEUROSCI.20-15-05709.2000

[82] Assis-de-lemos G, Moura-do-nascimento R, Amaral-do-nascimento M, Miceli AC, Vieira TCRG. Interactions between cytokines and the pathogenesis of prion diseases: Insights and implications. Brain Sciences. 2024;**14**(5):413. DOI: 10.3390/brainsci14050413

[83] de Melo ASLF, Lima JLD, Malta MCS, Marroquim NF, Moreira ÁR, de Almeida Ladeia I, Dos Santos Cardoso F, Gonçalves DB, Dutra BG, Dos Santos JCC. The role of microglia in prion diseases and possible therapeutic targets: A literature review. Prion. 2021;**15**(1):191–206. DOI: 10.1080/19336896.2021.1991771

[84] Carroll JA, Chesebro B. Neuroinflammation, microglia, and cell-association during prion disease. Viruses. 2019;**11**(1):65. DOI: 10.3390/v11010065

[85] Kinney JW, Bemiller SM, Murtishaw AS, Leisgang AM, Salazar AM, Lamb BT. Inflammation as a central mechanism in Alzheimer's disease. Alzheimer's & Dementia (New York, N.Y.). 2018;**4**:575–590. DOI: 10.1016/j.trci.2018.06.014

[86] Makarava N, Safadi T, Bocharova O, Mychko O, Pandit NP, Molesworth K, Baskakov IV et al. Reactive microglia partially envelop viable neurons in prion diseases. The Journal of Clinical Investigation. 2024;**134**(23):e181169

[87] Zhang W, Xiao D, Mao Q, et al. Role of neuroinflammation in neurodegeneration development. Signal Transduction and Targeted Therapy. 2023;**8**:267

[88] Wang Y, Hartmann K, Thies E, Mohammadi B, Altmeppen H, Sepulveda-Falla D, Krasemann S. Loss of homeostatic microglia signature in prion diseases. Cells. 2022;**11**(19):2948

[89] Moon JH, Hong JM, Park SY. Calcineurin activation by prion protein induces neurotoxicity via mitochondrial reactive oxygen species. Oxidative Medicine and Cellular Longevity. 2021;**2021**:5572129. DOI: 10.1155/2021/5572129

[90] Aguzzi A, Zhu C. Microglia in prion diseases. The Journal of Clinical Investigation. 2017;**127**(9):3230–3239

[91] Boje KM, Arora PK. Microglial-produced nitric oxide and reactive nitrogen oxides mediate neuronal cell death. Brain Research. 1992;**587**(2):250–256

[92] Simpson DSA, Oliver PL. ROS generation in microglia: Understanding oxidative stress and inflammation in neurodegenerative disease. Antioxidants (Basel, Switzerland). 2020;**9**(8):743. DOI: 10.3390/antiox9080743

[93] Bourgognon JM, Spiers JG, Robinson SW, Scheiblich H, Glynn P, Ortori C, Steinert JR et al. Inhibition of neuroinflammatory nitric oxide signaling suppresses glycation and prevents neuronal dysfunction in mouse prion disease. Proceedings of the National Academy of Sciences. 2021;**118**(10):e2009579118

[94] Moore S, Meschkat M, Ruhwedel T, et al. A role of oligodendrocytes in information

processing. Nature Communications. 2020;**11**:5497

[95] Bokulic Panichi L, Stanca S, Dolciotti C, Bongioanni P. The role of oligodendrocytes in neurodegenerative diseases: Unwrapping the layers. International Journal of Molecular Sciences. 2025;**26**(10):4623. DOI: 10.3390/ijms26104623

[96] Sponne I, Fifre A, Koziel V, Kriem B, Oster T, Olivier JL, Pillot T. Oligodendrocytes are susceptible to apoptotic cell death induced by prion protein-derived peptides. Glia. 2004;**47** (1):1–8

[97] Kirby L, Jin J, Cardona JG, Smith MD, Martin KA, Wang J, Strasburger H, Herbst L, Alexis M, Karnell J, Davidson T, Dutta R, Goverman J, Bergles D, Calabresi PA. Oligodendrocyte precursor cells present antigen and are cytotoxic targets in inflammatory demyelination. Nature Communications. 2019;**10** (1):3887. DOI: 10.1038/s41467-019-11638-3

[98] Dar NJ, Bhat JA, John U, Bhat SA. Neuroglia in neurodegeneration: Exploring glial dynamics in brain disorders. Neuroglia. 2024;**5**(4):488–504. DOI: 10.3390/neuroglia5040031

[99] Magni G, Riboldi B, Ceruti S. Human glial cells as innovative targets for the therapy of central nervous system pathologies. Cells. 2024;**13** (7):606. DOI: 10.3390/cells13070606

[100] Andreasson KI, Bachstetter AD, Colonna M, Ginhoux F, Holmes C, Lamb B, Van Eldik LJ, et al.. Targeting innate immunity for neurodegenerative disorders of the central nervous system. Cold Spring Harbor Perspectives in Biology. 2016;**138**(5):653–693

[101] Moussa N, Dayoub N. Exploring the role of COX-2 in Alzheimer's disease: Potential therapeutic implications of COX-2 inhibitors. Saudi Pharmaceutical Journal. 2023;**31** (9):101729. DOI: 10.1016/j.jsps.2023.101729

[102] PL M, EG M. NSAIDs and Alzheimer disease: Epidemiological, animal model and clinical studies. Neurobiology of Aging. 2007;**28** (5):639–647. DOI: 10.1016/j.neurobiolaging.2006.03.013

[103] Márquez Loza A, Elias V, Wong CP, Ho E, Bermudez M, Magnusson KR. Effects of ibuprofen on cognition and NMDA receptor subunit expression across aging. Neuroscience. 2017;**344**:276–292. DOI: 10.1016/j.neuroscience.2016.12.041

[104] Meinert ADAPTRG, L. C, McCaffrey LD, Breitner JC. Alzheimer's Disease Anti-inflammatory Prevention Trial: Design, methods, and baseline results. Alzheimer's & Dementia: The Journal of the Alzheimer's Association. 2009;**5**(2):93–104. DOI: 10.1016/j.jalz.2008.09.004

[105] Qin J, Ma Z, Chen X, Shu S. Microglia activation in central nervous system disorders: A review of recent mechanistic investigations and development efforts. Frontiers in Neurology. 2023;**14**:1103416. DOI: 10.3389/fneur.2023.1103416

[106] Shaftel SS, Carlson TJ, Olschowka JA, Kyrkanides S, Matousek SB, O'Banion MK. Chronic interleukin-1beta expression in mouse brain leads to leukocyte infiltration and neutrophil-independent blood brain barrier permeability without overt neurodegeneration. The Journal of Neuroscience: The Official Journal of

the Society for Neuroscience. 2007;**27**(35):9301–9309. DOI: 10.1523/JNEUROSCI.1418-07.2007

[107] Shaftel SS, Griffin WS, O'Banion MK. The role of interleukin-1 in neuroinflammation and Alzheimer disease: An evolving perspective. Journal of Neuroinflammation. 2008;**5**:7. DOI: 10.1186/1742-2094-5-7

[108] GuoYan L, ShuQin Z, HuiYang Q, MengYing C, HongWei R, Hong S. IL-8 and IL-1β in the cerebrospinal fluid of patient with Creutzfeldt-Jakob disease: A case report. Clinical Case Reports. 2025;**13**(5):e70508. DOI: 10.1002/ccr3.70508

[109] Onuska KM. The dual role of microglia in the progression of Alzheimer's disease. The Journal of Neuroscience: The Official Journal of the Society for Neuroscience. 2020;**40**(8):1608–1610. DOI: 10.1523/JNEUROSCI.2594-19.2020

[110] He C, Chen B, Yang H, Zhou X. The dual role of microglia in Alzheimer's disease: From immune regulation to pathological progression. Frontiers in Aging Neuroscience. 2025;**17**:1554398. DOI: 10.3389/fnagi.2025.15543

[111] Deming Y, Li Z, Benitez BA, Cruchaga C. Triggering receptor expressed on myeloid cells 2 (TREM2): A potential therapeutic target for Alzheimer disease? Expert Opinion on Therapeutic Targets. 2018;**22**(7):587–598. DOI: 10.1080/14728222.2018.1486823

[112] Qu W, Li L. Microglial TREM2 at the intersection of brain aging and Alzheimer's disease. The Neuroscientist: A Review Journal Bringing Neurobiology, Neurology and Psychiatry. 2023;**29**(3):302–316. DOI: 10.1177/10738584211040786

[113] Deczkowska A, Keren-Shaul H, Weiner A, Colonna M, Schwartz M, Amit I. Disease-associated microglia: A universal immune sensor of neurodegeneration. Cell. 2018;**173**(5):1073–1081

[114] Long H, Simmons A, Mayorga A, Burgess B, Nguyen T, Budda B, Rychkova A, Rhinn H, Tassi I, Ward M, Yeh F, Schwabe T, Paul R, Kenkare-Mitra S, Rosenthal A. Preclinical and first-in-human evaluation of AL002, a novel TREM2 agonistic antibody for Alzheimer's disease. Alzheimer's Research & Therapy. 2024;**16**(1):235. DOI: 10.1186/s13195-024-01599-1

[115] Chitu V, Gokhan Ş, Nandi S, Mehler MF, Stanley ER. Emerging roles for CSF-1 receptor and its ligands in the nervous system. Trends in Neurosciences. 2016;**39**(6):378–393. DOI: 10.1016/j.tins.2016.03.005

[116] Hu B, Duan S, Wang Z, Li X, Zhou Y, Zhang X, Zheng H et al. Insights into the role of CSF1R in the central nervous system and neurological disorders. Frontiers in Aging Neuroscience. 2021;**13**:789834

[117] De I, Nikodemova M, Steffen MD, Sokn E, Maklakova VI, Watters JJ, Collier LS. CSF1 overexpression has pleiotropic effects on microglia in vivo. Glia. 2014;**62**(12):1955–1967

[118] Henry RJ, Ritzel RM, Barrett JP, Doran SJ, Jiao Y, Leach JB, Szeto GL, Wu J, Stoica BA, Faden AI, Loane DJ. Microglial depletion with CSF1R inhibitor during chronic phase of experimental traumatic brain injury reduces neurodegeneration and neurological deficits. The Journal of

Neuroscience: The Official Journal of the Society for Neuroscience. 2020;**40**(14):2960–2974. DOI: 10.1523/JNEUROSCI.2402-19.2020

[119] Han J, Chitu V, Stanley ER, Wszolek ZK, Karrenbauer VD, Harris RA. Inhibition of colony stimulating factor-1 receptor (CSF-1R) as a potential therapeutic strategy for neurodegenerative diseases: Opportunities and challenges. Cellular and Molecular Life Sciences. 2022;**79**(4):219. DOI: 10.1007/s00018-022-04225-1

[120] Race B, Williams K, Baune C, Striebel JF, Long D, Thomas T, Lubke L, Chesebro B, Carroll JA. Microglia have limited influence on early prion pathogenesis, clearance, or replication. PloS One. 2022;**17**(10):e0276850. DOI: 10.1371/journal.pone.0276850

[121] Miao J, Ma H, Yang Y, Liao Y, Lin C, Zheng J, Yu M, Lan J. Microglia in Alzheimer's disease: Pathogenesis, mechanisms, and therapeutic potentials. Frontiers in Aging Neuroscience. 2023;**15**:1201982. DOI: 10.3389/fnagi.2023.1201982

[122] Kim K, Lee SG, Kegelman TP, et al. Role of excitatory amino acid transporter-2 (EAAT2) and glutamate in neurodegeneration: Opportunities for developing novel therapeutics. Journal of Cellular Physiology. 2011;**226**(10):2484–2493. DOI: 10.1002/jcp.22609

[123] Lee SG, Su ZZ, Emdad L, Gupta P, Sarkar D, Borjabad A, Volsky DJ, Fisher PB. Mechanism of ceftriaxone induction of excitatory amino acid transporter-2 expression and glutamate uptake in primary human astrocytes. Journal of Biological Chemistry. 2008;**283**(19):13116–13123. DOI: 10.1074/jbc.M707697200

[124] Fontana AC, Fox DP, Zoubroulis A, Mortensen OV, Raghupathi R. Neuroprotective effects of the glutamate transporter activator (R)-(-)-5-methyl-1-nicotinoyl-2-pyrazoline (MS-153) following traumatic brain injury in the adult rat. Journal of Neurotrauma. 2016;**33**(11):1073–1083. DOI: 10.1089/neu.2015.4079

[125] Kong Q, Chang LC, Takahashi K, Liu Q, Schulte DA, Lai L, Ibabao B, Lin Y, Stouffer N, Das Mukhopadhyay C, Xing X, Seyb KI, Cuny GD, Glicksman MA, Lin CL. Small-molecule activator of glutamate transporter EAAT2 translation provides neuroprotection. Journal of Clinical Investigation. 2014;**124**(3):1255–1267. DOI: 10.1172/JCI66163

[126] Weller ML, Stone IM, Goss A, Rau T, Rova C, Poulsen DJ. Selective overexpression of excitatory amino acid transporter 2 (EAAT2) in astrocytes enhances neuroprotection from moderate but not severe hypoxia-ischemia. Neuroscience. 2008;**155**(4):1204–1211. DOI: 10.1016/j.neuroscience.2008.05.059

[127] Jain M, Singh MK, Shyam H, Mishra A, Kumar S, Kumar A, Kushwaha J. Role of JAK/STAT in the neuroinflammation and its association with neurological disorders. Annals of Neurosciences. 2021;**28**(3-4):191–200

[128] Haim LB, Ceyzériat K, Carrillo-de Sauvage MA, Aubry F, Auregan G, Guillermier M, Escartin C et al. The JAK/STAT3 pathway is a common inducer of astrocyte reactivity in Alzheimer's and Huntington's diseases.

Journal of Neuroscience. 2015;**35**(6):2817–2829

[129] Reichenbach N, Delekate A, Plescher M, Schmitt F, Krauss S, Blank N, Halle A, Petzold GC. Inhibition of Stat3-mediated astrogliosis ameliorates pathology in an Alzheimer's disease model. EMBO Molecular Medicine. 2019;**11**(2):e9665. DOI: 10.15252/emmm.201809665

[130] Raible DJ, Frey LC, Brooks-Kayal AR. Effects of JAK2-STAT3 signaling after cerebral insults. Jak-stat. 2014;**3**(2):e29510. DOI: 10.4161/jkst.29510

[131] An JY, Pang HG, Huang TQ, Song JN, Li DD, Zhao YL, Ma XD. AG490 ameliorates early brain injury via inhibition of JAK2/STAT3-mediated regulation of HMGB1 in subarachnoid hemorrhage. Experimental and Therapeutic Medicine. 2018;**15**(2):1330–1338. DOI: 10.3892/etm.2017.5539

[132] Chen KS, Koubek EJ, Sakowski SA, Feldman EL. Stem cell therapeutics and gene therapy for neurologic disorders. Neurotherapeutics. 2024;**21**(4):e00427

[133] Kim SU, Lee HJ, Kim YB. Neural stem cell-based treatment for neurodegenerative diseases. Neuropathology: Official Journal of the Japanese Society of Neuropathology. 2013;**33**(5):491–504. DOI: 10.1111/neup.12020

[134] Wolfe CM, Fitz NF, Nam KN, Lefterov I, Koldamova R. The role of APOE and TREM2 in Alzheimer's disease-current understanding and perspectives. International Journal of Molecular Sciences. 2018;**20**(1):81. DOI: 10.3390/ijms20010081

[135] Lin YT, Seo J, Gao F, Feldman HM, Wen HL, Penney J, Cam HP, Gjoneska E, Raja WK, Cheng J, Rueda R, Kritskiy O, Abdurrob F, Peng Z, Milo B, Yu CJ, Elmsaouri S, Dey D, Ko T, Yankner BA, Tsai LH. APOE4 causes widespread molecular and cellular alterations associated with Alzheimer's disease phenotypes in human iPSC-derived brain cell types. Neuron. 2018;**98**(6):1141–1154.e7. Epub 2018 May 31. Erratum in: Neuron. 2018 Jun 27;98(6):1294. doi: 10.1016/j.neuron.2018.06.011. DOI: 10.1016/j.neuron.2018.05.008

[136] Teter B, Campagna J, Zhu C, McCauley GE, Spilman P, Kohn DB, John V (2024). Successful gene editing of apolipoprotein E4 to E3 in brain of Alzheimer model mice after a single IV Dose of Synthetic Exosome-Delivered CRISPR. bioRxiv, 2024–04

[137] Garcia-Reitboeck P, Phillips A, Piers TM, Villegas-Llerena C, Butler M, Mallach A, Pocock JM et al. Human induced pluripotent stem cell-derived microglia-like cells harboring TREM2 missense mutations show specific deficits in phagocytosis. Cell Reports. 2018;**24**(9):2300–2311

[138] Piers TM, Cosker K, Mallach A, Johnson GT, Guerreiro R, Hardy J, Pocock JM. A locked immunometabolic switch underlies TREM2 R47H loss of function in human iPSC-derived microglia. The FASEB Journal. 2020;**34**(2):2436–2450. DOI: 10.1096/fj.201902447R

[139] Hastings N, Kuan WL, Osborne A, Kotter MRN. Therapeutic potential of astrocyte transplantation. Cell Transplantation. 2022;**31**:9636897221105499. DOI: 10.1177/09636897221105499

[140] Krencik R, Weick J, Liu Y, et al. Specification of transplantable astroglial subtypes from human pluripotent stem cells. Nature Biotechnology. 2011;**29**:528–534

[141] Armijo E, Edwards G, Flores A, Vera J, Shahnawaz M, Moda F, Gonzalez C, Sanhueza M, Soto C. Induced pluripotent stem cell-derived neural precursors improve memory, synaptic and pathological abnormalities in a mouse model of Alzheimer's disease. Cells. 2021;**10**(7):1802. DOI: 10.3390/cells10071802

[142] Ifediora N, Canoll P, Hargus G. Human stem cell transplantation models of Alzheimer's disease. Frontiers in Aging Neuroscience. 2024;**16**:1354164. DOI: 10.3389/fnagi.2024.1354164

[143] Windrem MS, Schanz SJ, Zou L, Chandler-Militello D, Kuypers NJ, Nedergaard M, Goldman SA. Human glial progenitor cells effectively remyelinate the demyelinated adult brain. Cell Reports. 2020;**31**(7):107658

[144] Wang Y, Cella M, Mallinson K, Ulrich JD, Young KL, Robinette ML, Colonna M et al. TREM2 lipid sensing sustains the microglial response in an Alzheimer's disease model. Cell. 2015;**160**(6):1061–1071